Cancer
Overcome
by Diet

An
Alternative
to
Surgery

by
Louise Greenfield

Midwest Publishing Co.
Livonia, Michigan

Library of Congress Number: 86-061770

ISBN: 0-9617947-0-4

For information, address:
Midwest Publishing Co.
19970 Lathers Avenue
Livonia, Mich. 48152
U.S.A.

DEDICATIONS

To my husband, DAVID, who pointed the way to the diet, and then gave up meat and other foods to make it easier for me to prepare our daily meals.

To DR. JACK GOLDSTEIN, who devised the diet and saved me from mutilation.

To DR. ANNE SAMBORSKI, who gave me steady support and encouragement.

AND

To my readers — please bring an open mind to your reading of this book. Let me take you on an adventure into new ways of thinking about health and illness.

This book is the story of my personal struggle with cancer and the unique method I chose to overcome it. My book is not intended to replace the advice of your doctor.

Contents

ZIEGER OSTEOPATHIC HOSPITAL
BOTSFORD GENERAL HOSPITAL

DEPARTMENT OF

PATHOLOGY

TISSUE STUDY

Case No. 4768452

Room Amb.Surg.

Name Greenfield, Louise   Age 49   Sex f   SMWD   Race

Tissue Specimen(s) to be Examined   Right breast

Clinical Diagnosis   tumor

Exact Source of Biopsy

Requested 12-14- 19 7 Pr.   Mainster   Dr.   Knight
                                        Surgeon   Referring

Laboratory No. Sp. 77- B 60230   Dec 16, 1977

GROSS SPECIMEN: Submitted was a fibrofatty mass 4.5 x 3 x 2 cm. demonstrating
multiple cysts the largest 2.5 cm. in diameter, the cyst appears to be
containing a cloudy fluid.

MICROSCOPY: Sections taken of the mass demonstrated cystic disease whereby
there appear dilated cystic spaces as well as apocrine metaplasia. In some
areas the ducts appear to be lined by an epithelium which appears to be
hyperchromatic, the nuclei appear pleomorphic, bizarre mitotic figures
are seen scattered throughout. Within the lumen of these glandular structures
lined by this atypical epithelium appears to be necrotic debris. Infiltration
of this neoplasm into the associated fibrofatty stroma of the breast is
also identified. These features appear to be consistent with an infiltrating
ductal adenocarcinoma of the comedo cell type. This comedo infiltrating
ductal pattern seems to be scattered throughout the breast tissue submitted.

SUMMARY: A large breast biopsy demonstrated areas of cystic disease as well as an infiltrating adenocarcinoma of the breast, ductal, comedo cell type. The lesion appears to be multi-eccentric. Cellular atypia 1s of a Grade II.

DIAGNOSIS: Infiltrating ductal adenocarcinoma, comedo cell type (T0400-M8503)(.6)(A)

REPORT TO: MICHIGAN STATE CANCER CONTROL.

_____ D.O.
Pathologist

_____ D.O.
Director of Laboratories

CHAPTER I

A Chilling Diagnosis

It is said that a certain man lived to be 100 years old. When asked why he had lived so long, he replied that it had mostly to do with attitude towards life's happenings. He said, "Life is sweet if you know how to live it; otherwise it can be very bitter."

Life wasn't very sweet for me in 1977. Instead, it was full of stress and strain. I had a difficult job and a tough boss. I had two sons, the older of whom was behaving badly in college. I had a second husband who was hostile towards my sons. I was suffering from colitis and carried a persistent pain in my abdomen.

There didn't seem to be any relief in sight. Family counseling helped, but not enough. My boss got meaner by the day, which I couldn't understand since I was pleasant and efficient and got lots of work done. But then, he was mean to everyone in the department. I was trying desperately to keep my job because I needed the money to support my sons. Also, I wanted to work at least five more years so that I could lock in my pension benefits.

One day in November of 1977 I felt so dragged down by minor physical ailments that I went to my family doctor. That's when my life, already far from sweet, became doubly bitter.

As my doctor gave me a routine breast examination, his

face suddenly grew serious. Dr. Kane is a good doctor and a wonderful man—concerned, warm, caring, who answers your questions.

He said, "You have two small lumps here. I examine breasts all day long, and these are dangerous ones. I want you to have a mammogram."

I went to a lab and had the mammogram. When Dr. Kane got the results he called my husband and me into his office. He explained that the lumps were malignant and had to be removed. He went on to say, "As you know, I don't do surgery, so I am sending you to Dr. May. He is a good man who keeps up on all the latest university teachings."

My husband was stunned. As for myself, I was terrified of losing my breast and terrified of going into the hospital. My mother had died in a hospital at the age of thirty-five.

We went to see Dr. May. He read the mammogram, also, and agreed that an operation was necessary. I told him, very forcefully, to remove only the lumps, not the entire breast, no matter what he found. I wanted to come out of the operation and talk things over. It was my body and I wanted to participate in such a big decision.

I had heard of a few cases where the doctors had gone ahead and removed the entire breast and the poor woman woke up to find herself stripped of this part of her body. It was my opinion that this was colossal arrogance on the part of the doctors involved and I was determined this wouldn't happen to me.

The hospital I went into was a rather small one, but the care was excellent and they had the latest equipment there. Everyone treated me nicely, and I think this was probably due to the hospital being small. I had the lumpectomy on an out-patient basis. I was admitted at 9:00 A.M. and at 4:00 P.M. my husband, Dave, drove me home.

A few days later we went into Dr. May's office to have the incision checked. At that time Dr. May told me the lumps had been analyzed and he said the lab report stated the cancer cells were spreading. He advised an immediate modified mastectomy. I asked to see the lab report that he was holding in his hands.

He seemed a bit surprised, but gave it to me. There were the dreadful words, "an infiltrating adenocarcinoma of the breast" plus many technical words. At the bottom it said, "Report to: Michigan State Cancer Control." Now I was a statistic.

I told Dr. May I needed more time to make this decision. He became very angry. He pressed the intercom button and bellowed, "Send Mr. Greenfield in here."

Dave came in and Dr. May told him what the lab said and repeated his advice that I should have my right breast removed. My husband, bless his heart, took my side; he said we needed a few days to think it over.

The doctor let us go, reluctantly. "You are taking a terrible chance with this woman's life," he barked at us.

I looked at him, feeling like a stricken animal, and walked out of the room without saying another word.

I was thrown into a terrible state — it must have been pure terror. I felt as if I had one foot in the grave; I immediately thought that I must update my will. I wondered who would take care of my boys after I died. As their stepfather, Dave couldn't be expected to take care of them. Their natural father had remarried and I knew his new wife would not welcome two teenage boys, especially since her own son had just left home.

Another problem faced me at work. I had a strong, deep feeling that if I told my boss I had cancer I would be out of his department in a hurry, and maybe even out of the company. I needed my job — who doesn't? — and as I said before, I was trying to lock in my retirement benefits. I used my preexisting ailment, colitis, as an excuse. Colitis is inflammation of the intestines which causes gas, pain, and diarrhea. I controlled it with the drug bentyl, and a bland diet. To avoid mentioning my cancer, I told my boss my colitis was flaring up and that's why I had to take some time off.

A few days later Dr. May's office called and his secretary wanted to know when she could schedule the operation. Dave fended her off and a little later the surgeon himself called. I refused to talk to him; I was afraid he would push me into something I wasn't ready for. He insisted on speaking to Dave.

He told him that my operation must be done RIGHT AWAY. He said he kept in close touch with a big teaching hospital and he knew the latest "treatment of choice." This was a modified mastectomy, which removed only the breast, the small pectoral muscle, and the lymph nodes in the armpit. A radical mastectomy would remove all of those plus the large pectoral muscle, the absence of which makes it extremely difficult and painful to regain normal use of the arm. Dr. May implied how lucky I was that radical mastectomies were no longer used as a matter of course.

My husband told him firmly, "Not just yet, Doctor, we will let you know later."

That was the beginning of hell of earth for me. An experienced, knowledgeable doctor was telling me what to do, and I was refusing to follow his advice. What, then, was I to do?

For starters, we told Dr. May's office to send the slide to the University of Michigan lab for reading. The results were the same.

Back to square one. Again the question, what was I to do?

I don't recall shedding any tears during that time. This surprised me, I was so quick to weep at movies with sad endings. I do recall having great trouble sleeping. It was as if, when I closed my eyes, a brown fog dropped over me. After many restless nights I began saying the alphabet with flowers — aster, begonia, chrysanthemum, daffodil, etc. — and would repeat and repeat until I fell asleep.

We knew of Dr. Jack Goldstein, author of TRIUMPH OVER DISEASE BY FASTING AND NATURAL DIET. In this book—a marvelous book which reads like an adventure story—Dr. Goldstein, a podiatrist and nutritional consultant in Livonia, Michigan, tells how he cured himself of a devastating case of ulcerative colitis. He did it as the title says, through fasting and natural diet.

Since I was in such a state of sheer terror, I never even thought of him, even though he had been my own foot doctor for a number of years. Fortunately, my husband suggested we seek his advice. We called for an appointment, but it being near Christmas it would be a week before we could get in to see him. I began eating lots of raw fruits and nuts from the shell, since I knew from his book that raw foods helped cure him.

After a few days I thought, well, this wouldn't be too bad, apples and oranges and bananas have a nice taste. Little did I know what I was in for. It was going to be, Green Vegetables!

We went in for the consultation. Dr. Goldstein is a tall, nicely built man with a ready laugh and quick sense of humor. He took my medical history, including the details of my diagnosis and operation. He said it was to my benefit I had limited my medical treatment to a lumpectomy. He said that radiation and chemotherapy are harmful to the body because these things kill normal cells as well as cancerous ones.

"Then why do they give these treatments to people?" I asked.

"Because they hope the normal cells will survive in great enough numbers to save the patients. It's the only thing they know to do."

"My big question is this, Doctor. I read your book, so I understand why raw vegetables cured your colitis. But cancer is so much worse. How can raw food cure cancer?"

"I can tell how upset you are. It's a complex subject and if I told you the details, five minutes later you wouldn't remember. But basically, cancer is caused by things going wrong inside the body, and raw vegetables have vitamins and minerals in perfect balance. When taken as liquid the vitamins and minerals go right into the blood stream and thus allow the body to heal itself."

"But bodies don't heal themselves," I said.

He smiled. "What do you think heals you?"

"Why, the doctor and the drugs he gives you."

He smiled again. "I thought you read my book."

"Yes, but this is cancer."

"In the last analysis, it is your body that heals itself. Take my word for it, until you are able to do your own studying. Now with your health history in mind, I'm going to write out a diet for you."

He wrote busily for long minutes while I stared at the field of daisies in the picture hanging on the wall behind him. I had seen this picture many times before, when I had visited his office previously for my foot treatments. There's a young child picking daisies in the field. That young child had his life ahead of him, but for all I knew, my life was over.

Dr. Goldstein handed me the diet. He explained that it would correct the imbalance in my system and get it to the point where my immune system could kick in and vanquish the cancer.

I didn't really understand what he was saying, but from having read his book, I knew he was a brilliant chemist. And from having been his foot patient for ten years, I knew he was an honest man who never tried to talk you into anything you didn't need. So I decided I would put myself in his hands and trust in his word.

He also told us how to prepare the foods, where to buy them, what sort of juicer and blender to buy. Basically my diet would comprise raw vegetable juice, raw blended salad, whole fruits, raw milk cheese, raw unsalted nuts, and certain legumes and other foods that were naturally full of B-17, the anti-cancer vitamin.

We went home. I already had a heavy-duty blender which I could use to make the blended salad, but we needed the juice extractor. Dave went out and bought one. It is an Oster centrifugal juicer, and never gave me a minute's trouble. I'm still using it every day.

This was in late December, 1977. I stayed home and returned to work on January 11th. Dave and I worked in the same building and rode together in the same car. This saved on gas, but sometimes it was bad for marital harmony. If there'd been a squabble at home, it carried over into the car. We had developed the habit of not talking during these morning rides.

After the cancer, however, there was truly nothing to talk about. There was one thought — one fear, actually — uppermost in both our minds — would I die of it? How soon? With how much pain? Neither of us could talk about it.

Dave's true colors began to come out. Before this he was something of a stinker. He used to pick at my sons and criticize me, but gradually he changed. He became loving, helpful, and devoted. I told him I couldn't cook meat and other foods for him and the boys and then not eat some myself, it was just too cruel.

So he went on the diet with me. For this, I owe him a very great deal. I know of one woman who attempted this same diet but her husband made such a fuss about having his meat that he quite sabotaged her efforts to eat differently.

For the first several months that I was on the diet, I was weak from the radical change in food. In the mornings Dave made the raw juice and the blended salad and put them into thermos bottles to take to work. He also cleaned out these appliances while I dressed and made the bed. His true colors turned out to be true blue for loyalty and loving pink for devotion. It may sound sentimental, but I can truthfully say that my brush with cancer improved our relationship.

My colitis gave me many problems with maintaining the diet exactly as written. So many of the foods gave me raging gas in the intestines. In addition, Dr. Goldstein told me it was very important that I did not put any chemicals into my system. This meant no medicines, no sleeping pills, no tranquilizers, no antibiotics, no aspirin — all those wonderful, handy drugs which give us a quick fix and permit us to go back to work without missing any time. This meant no more bentyl to soothe my irritable colon.

At times my system was so bloated with gas I could have floated away. But the gas was stuck inside me; I could never seem to pass it out. I had a persistent ache in my abdomen, low on the right side. This made it difficult to continue working. As an accountant, I sat all day long. Sitting for hours was uncomfortable, sometimes painful, and with my boss cracking the whip the way he was, I didn't dare get up and move around too often.

I wondered whether to tell my sons. My first impulse was not to tell them, because I didn't want them to be scared and worried. Accordingly, I concealed it for a while, but soon it became impossible to go on with the charade. I felt so weak, so totally awful that I could not summon up the energy to act as if everything was normal. So I told them. It didn't take too many words, and I haven't the faintest recollection of what I said. But the deed was done and as time went on I was to learn what the news of my cancer did to them.

My younger boy, Stuart, smothered over his feelings and school studies became his security blanket. He had already been a good student, now he became an excellent one. He studied constantly, dropped the swim team and debate team, and wouldn't socialize except with a buddy who was another serious student.

My older boy, Keith, obviously felt rattled and insecure.

He had been a difficult child at various times and now, a freshman at college, he simply went wild. He neglected his studies and kept dropping classes. He thought he was a genius who didn't have to obey the rules. He was a genius at one thing—he was a natural-born writer, just like a young Hemingway, and in addition to marvelous short stories, had written three excellent one-act plays. His high school drama teacher, a tough grader, thought highly of him.

At college, however, he was a small frog in a big puddle. No one gave him any recognition and this went down hard. Then, for his mother to be given a cancer diagnosis was too much for him to handle.

There was nothing I could do for him. He was away from home, and when he came home on vacations wouldn't talk to me. I was in such bad shape myself, that even had I known how to help him, I couldn't have done anything. He badgered me for money and luxury items and if he didn't get them his behavior worsened.

If I could have followed Dr. Goldstein's diet to the letter, it would have been easier. But because of my colitis, often I had to omit some of the legumes and protein. The nuts, in particular, were hard on my system, no matter how long and carefully I chewed them. Without enough protein, I became weak and stayed that way.

Earlier, when I made it clear to the surgeon, Dr. May, that I was not going to submit to the mastectomy, the issue came up of when I would return to work. He had to sign the release, inserting the date for return. When he realized I was not going to do it his way, he was clearly very angry. When I asked him to fill out the form, I mentioned the return date.

Because Dr. May was angry with me for refusing the operation, he told me to set the date instead of setting it himself. So I took a wild guess and said, "January 11th," and this is what he filled in. Later I was to realize that staying home for three weeks wasn't long enough to regain my strength. Therefore I wasn't strong enough and my early return left me weak for a long time.

This, plus not being able to tolerate enough protein, kept me in a weakened condition. Also, Dr. G's diet was two-pronged — eliminative and nutritive. That means toxins were being passed out, and my body went through many difficult spells which I later realized were "Healing Crises." I felt faint, weak, and it was difficult to concentrate.

At work, as an export accountant, I had to check details of foreign bank papers and shipping documents. I had to balance between $2 million and $4 million in accounts every month. This was a big responsibility, and I needed lots of energy, not less.

Another thing about this diet, I missed HOT foods. I never realized before what a dependence we all have on hot food — what a comfort it is. I would think and think and finally come up with something that Dr. G might allow. I'd call him up and ask, but he'd say no. I had to change the chemical balance in my body, he said, and cooked foods were DEAD FOODS and I couldn't have any. I couldn't have toast, even if it was made from unchemicalized bread, and I couldn't have hot tea, even if made from herbs.

These restrictions lasted four months. After that time (he was probably tired of my begging) Dr. G said I could have steamed vegetables. I still remember sitting down to my first hot food — a baked potato. It had no salt, no butter, no sour cream and chives — but it was heavenly. I told my family, don't bother me while I eat this wonderful thing on my plate.

I have been asked if I missed ordinary foods. Yes, I did. I can still recall the first time after my illness when I resumed the marketing. It was my habit to go on Tuesday right after work. I had my list, and, as usual, it included foods for the rest of my family. As I went up and down the aisles, seeing all the items I couldn't have — hot dogs, salami, steak, potato chips, cheese — I felt horrible. As I looked at the labels on prepared items and realized almost everything had chemicals, additives, and colorings in it and in the future would remain off my diet, I felt even worse. By the time I got halfway through the store, surrounded on all sides by shelves and shelves of foods I couldn't have, I could have beat my head on the wall, right there in front of all the other customers.

I told Dave about my experience and asked him to take over the grocery shopping. He readily agreed, and it was about four years before I went into a super market again. When I returned, it was the same as before—lots of food I couldn't have—most of it processed, packaged, and adulterated with chemicals of all sorts.

In October of 1984 I read a review of a new book about the food industry. It said $400 billion is spent on food in this country, but the farmer gets only 25 per cent of that. An executive for one of the biggest food companies was heard to bewail the fact that, with the general concern over cholesterol and not gaining too much weight, food consumption had leveled off and he moaned, "There are only so many stomachs." So how does the food industry respond to this problem? They come up with new products which process the food even MORE, so that they can charge more.

I cannot give the book a personal recommendation, as I have not read it, but it sounds very interesting. The title is: FAT OF THE LAND, by Fred Powledge. He also answers the interesting question: Why don't tomatoes have flavor any more?

The year 1978 crept by. My boss became dissatisfied with the amount of work I was producing. As I mentioned previously, I kept my cancer a secret at work. When they wanted to know about my operation, I told them it was for my colitis. My boss began nagging me to do more work. As time went by, it got so bad that I went to Central Personnel and asked them to intercede.

They came out and investigated and decided in my favor.

They told my boss to leave me alone. And he did. But his boss, the department manager — let's call him Mr. Peabody — was very upset that I had brought unfavorable attention to his department, and from then on, it was worse. I may have won the battle, but I lost the war, and Mr. Peabody was going to see to it.

Sometime earlier, a very pretty young woman had been hired as secretary in our department. She was hired in as a grade 2. My boss — let's call him Mr. Hamm — was bewitched by this cute young thing. Suffering as I was, I never noticed his attraction to her. He wanted to be nice to her. He wanted to do this by edging me out and giving her my job, which was two grades higher. But there was a little problem. Central Personnel had told him to stop persecuting me. So what could he do? Well, Mr. Hamm was a brilliant fellow, and he thought of something. He began sandbagging me — withholding my work and making it look like I was incompetent, by swamping my desk with paper as weekly deadlines neared.

When he spoke to me, he was sweet as honey and I never suspected a thing. I was working as best I could, but could never keep up and was beginning to doubt my abilities. I began to fear I would lose my job. This all added up to stress, and Dr. G's diet began to fail me. I'd call him, and he would reply, "I can give you the best diet in the world, but if you have too much continuing stress in your life, my diet won't do any good."

At that time I knew nothing about stress. I couldn't understand what he was telling me. To me, stress was something other people had, mostly top drawer business executives who were responsible for entire companies.

My older son, Keith, began acting up even worse. He'd dropped out of college and had come home. He slept all day, ran around with his buddies all night, and was generally uncooperative. Dave reacted to his behavior with great hostility. I was about to come apart at the seams.

All I could think of was working a few more years so I could lock in my retirement benefits, and save up for Stuart's college expenses.

The day of January 19, 1979 dawned. It was a wintry day. There was an average cover of snow on the ground. When I reported for work, Mr. Hamm called me into his office first thing. He handed me this big stack of work, and I couldn't imagine where he'd gotten it. It was enough for two days at least, if I worked at top speed.

He said sweetly, "Louise, you know you haven't been doing enough work. Here, see if you can get this done today. Show me what you can do. I think you can do it if you really try."

I took the pile to my desk and stared at it. I knew it was humanly impossible to do it in one day, even if I felt tip-top, which I didn't. But suddenly I thought, "I'll show that son of a bitch, I'll work like hell and see how much I can get done."

So I did. I worked like a fiend all day. I surprised myself by getting about three-fourths of it finished.

But at a terrible price. During the last three hours of the afternoon I had a dreadful pain in my breast. As I drove home with Dave, I had nothing to say. My mind was burned out. He asked what was wrong; with great effort I managed to tell him about the trick Mr. Hamm had played on me. I finished up by saying, "I don't think I will ever go back there again."

Dave said, "You don't have to go back, we can get along without their money."

And I never did.

CHAPTER II

Intimate Thoughts of a Cancer Patient

I have been a writer most of my life. I began at the age of eight, when I wrote a story about two little orphan sisters who had been sent to live with their grandmother. This was a thin disguise of my own life, except that I had no sister. (I had had a baby sister when I was six; my mother contracted double pneumonia, miscarried, and they both died.)

At school, I always did well in composition class. At twelve, I began a novel. It was another thin disguise, this time of GONE WITH THE WIND, my favorite book during my teen years.

When I graduated from college I wanted to become a college professor and novelist. I needed a Master of Arts degree in English. I began working on it, but I couldn't earn enough money to complete it. At that time the social pressures to marry and have children were very strong, and besides, I had to earn a living. I put my writing ambitions aside for the most part, went to work and got married. They always say a housewife can write on the side, but it doesn't always work out, especially when your first child is hyperactive, as mine was. But my desire to write was always in the back of my mind, and occasionally I would take a writing course and practice for the time ahead when I might be able to resume.

14

Fledgling writers are often advised to keep journals so they can gain practice, and to capture feelings when they are strongest. And so, periodically, I have kept journals. I want to share with you some of the things I wrote down after I learned I had cancer. This portion of my journal begins . . .

January 9, 1978 It is three weeks since I was told I have cancer. How do I cope with it? Much of the time I cannot; I cannot think of it directly. When I do, I either think in terms of getting my affairs in order, or why me? Why me? I don't smoke; I don't work in industry, supposedly two of the biggest causes of cancer. For about seven years I have omitted beef from my diet and I have, to some extent, avoided junk foods. Why me? What have I done?

And the worse thing of all, I haven't yet done what I want to do in this world. A few more years and my sons will be educated, and then I was planning to return to my writing and produce a book and get it published. A novel, or a book of my poems, or a non-fiction book — any kind of book, to share my hard-won wisdom with others, to leave some worthwhile reminder of myself on this earth. To finally gain the recognition and approval I have yearned for, for as many years as I can remember.

And now, my life is up for grabs. I may live, and I may not. On which basis do I plan what remains?

I have many ancestors who are long-lived — some lived to be over one hundred years old. Those who died young usually died of accidents. I had planned on living till at least eighty. After educating my boys, I had thought I would have twenty or thirty years to, at long last, do what I wanted to do for myself.

I cannot face the reality of dying. Whenever I try, I turn into a slobbering jelly of self-pity. I shall have to pretend that I am going to live.

Here it is, two o'clock in the afternoon, and I have at long last forced myself to shower and get dressed. Now that I have made up my face, I feel better. I feel as if I might live out this day, after all. One day at a time, perhaps that is my answer.

January 28, 1978 Last night, this is what I said to Dave. You know, honey, there are times when I want to talk to you about how I feel, but I can sense that you don't want to talk about it. That makes it hard for me. So I'm going to talk, whether you want to listen or not. Like tonight, when I was carefully flossing my teeth I thought suddenly, why am I bothering about my teeth? I have a far more serious problem. I may not even be here a year from now, who cares about teeth?

Then I try to think about it, but it slips away. Sometimes I think of the boys, and I feel so bad I may not be here to see them grow up. That I won't finish my job with them.

Other times I think about finding the lump, having the operation, the doctor telling me it was malignant, and all these things seem unreal. I can't believe they actually happened. I know they did, but they slip and slide away from me.

Sometimes I think about this freaky diet I am on and it is so boring and monotonous I would rather be dead than eat this way the rest of my life.

I think of the trip we took to Amsterdam and the wonderful veal dishes they cook over there. I think of how good sex used to be for us. And now, there's nothing. No comfort, no pleasure, no hope.

Then, Dave said, now it's my turn. We will go to Amsterdam again, and we will have great sex again, and you will get used to this diet, one day you will love it.

This last remark made me laugh. And he hugged me and it was okay for a while.

February 14, 1978 I thought I had so much time!

February 19, 1978 My memory cuts in and out like a computer without enough power. I kept thinking I must send in that monthly deposit for my sons' savings account for college, and I delayed it so long the month is gone; I decided to mail it in tomorrow with the next month's deposit. Today I received a copy of my receipted deposit slip from the bank. I had mailed it in and I can't remember doing any of it — writing the check or addressing the envelope or stamping it or anything else.

A few nights ago we went to see South Pacific at the Fisher Theatre. A stage show! I was thrilled to be attending. Then, once there, for the first half I was very uncomfortable with the format. Such tiny faces on the actors! I had grown used to big faces on the television screen. As the play went on, I hated it. I hated seeing those tight-skinned, young, agile bodies tossing themselves about the stage. And the revolting love theme — Garbage! I need someone young and smiling, sang the hero. Implying his life was empty and marrying this young nurse would fix things up. Oh yes, everyone wants company, affection, closeness — but why are there always fangs and thorns buried in our relationships? I went away hating the play.

Keith was home for the weekend, sniping at me, trying to hook me into the old games we used to play. Hope he does go to California to try for a film career. The day he leaves will be the happiest day of my life.

March, 1978 Dave is always sniping about Keith, whether he is here or not. Such jealousy. I've been to the lawyer and redone my will. I'm leaving my few pennies to the boys. Dave has plenty of dollars, he doesn't need mine, he's the executive, not me.

I had to ask my ex-husband to be guardian for under-age Stuart. He said yes. There's insurance on me at work; if I die as a full-time employee, I will be worth more dead than alive. What a grisly thought. Gives me a creepy feeling.

April, 1978 I am so tense. Mr. Hamm is cracking the whip at work. Keith is due home soon. Oh, how I wish I could take a tranquilizer. But Dr. G says, don't put any chemicals in your system.

May, 1978 I am so tired all the time. I can't concentrate. Maybe Mr. Hamm is right. Maybe I have turned into a lousy worker. But I try so hard. Next month is Dave's Army Reunion. He always expects me to go. Where will I find the strength? I'll need a new dress for the banquet; I'm so skinny I can't wear anything I have.

June 23, 1978 We are in Milwaukee for the Reunion. I am being bright and cheerful and pleasant, but oh, at what cost. After the banquet, on the final evening, did I have a bad night. We tried to make love and it flopped. Then we had a terrible confrontation. No, that makes it sound like we fought; rather, we talked about our gut feelings. He told me he still loves me but I get in these strange moods and he's afraid that if he approaches me for sex, I might feel worse. I cried and carried on and mentioned suicide, and said that I'd had a serious brush with it one time and, being without relatives, for many years took care to be a member of a church so I could call on the minister in the middle of the night if I ever felt like doing it again. I told him I felt my life was nothing but shit. He looked surprised. He knows I always avoid bad words like that. As a writer, with thousands of words at my command, I should not need to use vulgar words.

I mentioned the garbage at work, with Mr. Hamm trying to frame me, my bad feelings because Keith left home. I wanted him to leave, but as soon as he did, I felt guilty. I asked Dave, do you think it is fun to have cancer? To be forty-nine years old and never have done what you wanted to do? And then get cancer? To have this writing talent that is more like a disease than anything else? That you haven't been able to accomplish anything with, other than publish a few articles and stories? Can you think of any other word that puts fear into a person's heart like the word cancer does?

I was reading in the book, DANIEL MARTIN, where its

author says all writing is trying to deal with problems in the past and present. I don't quite understand that, but I do have a serious problem with my writing, and that's getting enough time for it.

It was so hard to talk. Dave said some comforting things, but I can't remember them. But at the end of it all, he hugged me close and said, I love you, I want you to know that. I said, I want to love you. He said, No, you don't, I'm a bastard toward your kids.

I went into a spasm. My body doubled up and I began hitting myself on the forehead and smashing my knees against the wall.

July, about a month later Though that was a very bad spell, it did me a lot of good. Apparently I unloaded a lot of bad feelings that were bothering me at gut level. It brought Dave and me closer. Exactly how, I don't know. But later he said he had changed toward Keith and if he had to come home — if he couldn't get a start in Hollywood — it would be okay now.

I suddenly realize, Dave has been good to me, in one big way. He has not rejected me sexually because of the cancer thing. Of course, I am not mutilated. Thanks to Dr. Goldstein's diet, I still have TWO BREASTS. The scar is small; it lies in a crescent just above my nipple and is not noticeable. There is a slight depression there, but not very bad.

August 1, 1978 Pete Rose is a ball player for the Cincinnati Reds. Dave loves baseball, and I have been hearing a lot about Pete Rose these days. Pete has gotten 44 hits in a row, beating the 36 hits in a row record in the National League by Tommy Holmes about twenty years ago. When Pete got 44 hits in a row, they were playing in Atlanta and he got a standing ovation. Now get this. An usherette was sent, by the **opposing** team, onto the field to present him with a bouquet of roses — 44 of them — one for each hit.

I got all broken up when I watched that presentation of

roses. When someone does something kind or thoughtful, something they don't **have** to do — it literally tears me apart. Does seeing kindness done remind me of the kindness I didn't get as a child? I don't know; but seeing Pete Rose get his roses caused such a reaction I had to leave the room.

New topic. Mr. Hamm got so nasty I called Central Personnel and asked them to investigate. They did, and they found him in the wrong, and told him to leave me alone. I hope he does. Oh, how I want to get my ten years in, so that I will have my own old-age pension. Maybe now I will have a chance.

August 4, 1978 This morning I was taking a shower. My hand passed across my left breast and there was a sharp pain above the nipple. I brought my hand back. A new lump, on the other breast. It had a square corner and was hard. Cancer again. More nightmare. First, terrible anger, mixed with frantic denial. Followed shortly by bitterness and cynicism. And a frightful hatred for every healthy person who crosses my path. Every now and then the sudden crying spell. Later the desperate feeling my life had turned into an absolute hell and the wild impulse to kill myself and end the fear and uncertainty once and for all.

I began thinking, what caused this lump? Decided it may have been because I took valium and bentyl for about two weeks. I took them because my depression was getting too suicidal. Suicide is a terrible thing within a family. I know of one case where the father did it and his teenage daughter was messed up forever. Also my discipline faltered. I bent my diet a little, eating a few too many dead foods and foods with additives. What would Dr. G say? Probably, I have told you the right way, why do you do wrong? But no, he is a kind man, he wouldn't reproach me.

August 12, 1978 I stopped the tranquilizers and observed the raw diet very carefully. Four days later the lump was almost gone. Seven days later, completely gone.

Did not dare to feel relief.

But I know now, I must not dare to stray from the diet. It is tough to observe, but the results of breaking it are too severe.

September 13, 1978 That lump went away. Now I find a new one. I have kept my diet, this one must be caused by tension. Tried to talk to Dave about it — I had concealed the one last month — but he wouldn't listen. I was furious. A lousy job, a gross husband, and a rotten kid, no wonder my stomach is tied up in knots.

September 15, 1978 Keith is back home. Dave is being nice. Keith went to Dr. Kane about a muscle problem and Dr. Kane said, your mother may think I'm mad at her because she wouldn't have surgery, but I'm not. I think about her a lot.

I was so surprised. Thought he had forgotten me long ago. Heart-warming to know someone is thinking about me. He always was a nice man and I thought well of him.

Late September, 1978 Went to a cancer nutrition seminar sponsored by the Foundation for Alternative Cancer Therapies. Mrs. Ruth Sackman, who runs the group, gave a speech and then asked for questions. Someone in the audience asked her **why** she was concerned with cancer, since she didn't have it herself. Mrs. Sackman bowed her head and paused for long moments. Finally she managed to speak, but her voice broke while she was doing so. She said that her daughter had died of cancer at a young age, suffering horribly from conventional treatment. Mrs. Sackman thought to herself, there must be some other way, and began investigating. She did find several other ways, and she wanted people to know there were **alternatives** to conventional medical treatment.

This seminar was a day-long thing on Saturday, with about eight speakers, and I took as many notes as I could, but it was so new a lot of it went right over my head. But one thing they kept saying was that cancer patients must not have stress in their daily lives.

When I stood in line at lunch, two ladies struck up a conversation with me.

One of them asked, "What is your interest in coming here?"

And I said, quite openly, "I am a cancer patient, and I took an alternative route, and I have survived—so far." I can't tell you what a relief that was to say it openly. Maybe I made a mistake, deciding not to tell about it at work. I might have lost my job, but I might have saved myself a lot of aggravation.

October 1, 1978 Read through my diary and was amazed I had written nothing about the trouble with Keith since his return from California. Too painful, I guess. Still too painful. Will put down a few words. He was in a Catch-22 situation. He couldn't find a job in California because he was camping and didn't have a local address. He couldn't get a local address because he didn't have a job.

When he first came back, he seemed a little grown up. But then he started playing Kid to my Mom. Wanting everything. Dave began bugging him to get a job, but he preferred to lie around. And so on, and so on.

March, 1979 Keith went back to college. What a relief. But also a worry. Is he going to buckle down and work? That's the question.

July, 1979 Am getting some pleasure out of working in the yard. Can't work for very long, my stamina is shot. But I enjoy working on my roses very much. They are one thing that don't betray me. Stuart graduated from high school in June. U of M has accepted him. Bills, bills, bills . . .

October, 1979 I have this fantasy of my life being peaceful, quiet and tension free. I don't expect happiness or riches, but oh, peace and quiet would be ideal.

Late October, 1979 More good news, ha! Dave's mother,

Vera, is ill. She has terrible pains in jaw and neck, she won't eat, she's in the hospital. She looks whiter than the sheets on her bed. Mr. Hamm is bugging me again. I feel so powerless. Keith dropped out of college. Vera came to live with us. Keith is fixing her meals and looking after her during the day. Oddly enough, he is doing a good job.

Early December, 1979 Keith has slipped. One day he called me at work and abused me over the phone. It's an open office and Ray, one of the accountants, overheard my end of the conversation. After I hung up he and I talked, and he made some good suggestions. He said, prepare for a separation in your mind, ask his dad for suggestions, try to have it amicable if possible, because if he goes away and you never hear from him, the uncertainty will be worse. Good advice. Nice guy.

I called my ex-husband, Dick. We met and I laid all the cards on the table, the moods, the bizarre behavior. He says he will help. Thank the Dear Lord.

Later December, 1979 Dick has talked to Keith and a target date has been set. I will let him take his clothes, his car, his typewriter, and I will give him $200 for a stake.

Later December, 1979 He is gone. The final scene was nastier than anything I could have dreamed. He is gone, but Vera is here. Just what I need. Someone else to take care of. When is my turn going to come?

CHAPTER III

Effects of Raw Diet

Vera was sent home with packets of medicine. They were giving her a total of twenty pills a day. She acted like a zombie. Really, a zombie! She moved stiffly, didn't talk, didn't read the paper. She never got dressed, just stayed in her robe, and sat motionless on a chair. She fed and toileted herself, period. Her skin was a pasty gray.

Her medical doctor said she had tic douloureux, that a pinched nerve in her neck was causing the pain. He said she needed many pills, first because she needed her usual heart and diuretic pills, then pain-killers which caused side effects which had to be treated with additional pills, which caused more side effects, which then had to be treated with additional pills.

We were aghast at what it added up to — twenty pills a day! We reasoned that if something were wrong with her neck, a carload of medication wouldn't cure it, but perhaps chiropractic care would.

She was 80 years old, and luckily our family chiropractor was willing to take her on. We took her for adjustments three times a week for six months, then twice a week for almost two years. Her doctor was Dr. Tony LaFramboise of Livonia. He is a fine gentleman with courtly manners, and there are no words to describe how gentle he was in his adjustments of her. Vera fell quite in love with him.

Dr. Tony had a heart attack in 1984 and has retired, and his retirement is a great loss to his profession. His son, Dr. Dan LaFramboise, continues in his footsteps. Dr. Dan has wonderful teaching abilities and is often asked to lecture.

To return to Vera. Since I was controlling my cancer without drugs, we took a very suspicious view of all the pills she was taking. Dr. Tony suggested we cut them back very gradually.

We followed his advice, and she began to improve. Her appetite perked up, her color returned. Within four months she was getting dressed every morning, putting on lipstick, fussing with her hair, and reading the paper. After six months, at which point we had cut her pills down to two a day (a heart pill and a diuretic) she was good as new. She was making afghans, cooking her own dinner, watching baseball games, keeping the box scores, reading the paper and making comments about current news stories.

When she attained good health, her personality came out. She proved to be charming and agreeable. It was like having a big baby around, she laughed at things I had stopped laughing at years ago. She was thrilled with every little thing you did for her.

Thinking about her improvement, and being sure that cutting down on her drugs was part of the reason, Dave and I began studying the subject.

The one ongoing problem Vera continued to have was pains in her legs at night due to poor circulation. Dave focused his studies on supplements and vitamins and came up with a regimen that eased her problem to a great degree. He was proving to be a very devoted son. At night when she moaned and groaned he would wake up and dash into her room to see how he could help her. I didn't wake up. She was not **MY** mother and he had not been a father to my boys, he hadn't even been a friend. Let him live up to **HIS** responsibilities, that was my thinking.

Don't misunderstand, please. I wasn't nasty to her, or unfeeling, and I was pleasant to her as I shared in her care during the day. But I was ill myself, with cancer and colitis and bad nerves. I could not be expected to get up at night with someone who wasn't of my own blood.

By the time Vera got on her feet, I had been off work for six months. I was on medical leave, but it was a very big question mark whether I would ever return. I was weak most of the time. I tired easily. Going out in the cold in wintertime dragged me down into the pits. Though I was avoiding the disfigurement of mastectomy and the pain and nausea of chemotherapy, I still occasionally found a new lump and wondered if I were doing the right thing. But I couldn't bear to think about it too long. I was **NOT** going to be mutilated, I was going to die the way God made me, and that was it.

I missed the girls at work. Though I worked for a very large firm, the division I worked for occupied only one floor, and there was a total of about 130 people there. Thirty of these were girls. We took our work breaks in two different shifts, so to speak, at mid-morning and mid-afternoon.

I worked in that place eight years and four months, and during that length of time, seeing the same girls twice a day, we all grew rather close. They were all nice women; we all got along well. There was one exception, a very catty woman who made lots of trouble by telling tales, but even the men couldn't stand her and managed to get rid of her. I had grown to feel that these girls were like sisters, and I, who had never known the affection of mother or sister, simply loved the feeling. I thought fondly of them, and this caused me fresh despair, because I knew I could never go back there, even if I ever got strong again. I could never again work within sight of Mr. Hamm or Mr. Peabody.

Dr. Goldstein had told me, many times, "You must get rid of the stress in your life," and those two men spelled stress and nothing else.

I also missed my paycheck. When I'd been elevated to my grade 4 job, that of Documentation Clerk in Export Finance, I'd received a hefty pay raise. In staying on that job three years, I'd had two merit increases, and for a woman I was making very good money. My ex-husband, though he always had a job, did not at this point in time have a good one, and could not help with the boys' education. Keith was out of the picture, but Stuart was going to the University of Michigan and I needed big money for that.

But, being home on sick leave, my pay was cut in half. There was no withholding, so my check was almost as big, but at the end of the year I had to pay taxes, so I set aside the necessary amount. Also, being on sick leave, I could no longer contribute to the stock savings plan, and thus could not build up my savings in that manner. I worried constantly about whether I would be able to fulfill my obligation to Stuart.

So, though some stress was eliminated by quitting, new stresses slipped in — missing my wonderful "sisters" at work, and worrying if I could put Stuart through the university. His grades were excellent, and he deserved the chance. Also, my father had educated me, so I owed it to the next generation to pass that benefit on.

A friend of mine (one of the few I told about my cancer) suggested I let Stuart work his way through. Well, I'd tried to work my way through graduate school and knew how tough it was. She suggested scholarships. I checked that out and found that because I was married to Dave, because his income appeared on our tax return, Stuart did not qualify.

So, despite being away from work, things were not that much better, though my diet had been liberalized little by little. I could have hot foods (mostly vegetables) and could eat chicken (raised without hormones) and fish.

Poor Dr. Goldstein! I really bent his ear over the phone. Those first few months I called him frequently with questions about the diet — the whys, and hows, but mostly requests for things that were not on his diet — vegetables he had not listed, and why no salad dressing, and why not this or that (hot) item.

He was unfailingly cheerful and always took the time to explain things to me. This whole way of life was so different that many times I could not understand things the first few times he explained them.

One of the most remarkable things the diet did for me involves a delicate matter, but it is a crucial one, so I must mention it. I have to back up a little to explain it.

Most of my life I never had trouble with constipation, except during pregnancy. When the colitis struck, back in 1976, at first I had diarrhea. As soon as Dr. Kane put me on medication the diarrhea cleared up. He also suggested a bland diet. This diet of cooked, smooth foods gave me constipation, which became an ongoing problem.

After I went on Dr. G's diet, this changed. I kept a brief diary of my reactions to the raw diet, and I'm going to repeat it here, exactly the way I jotted it down.

RAW DIARY

Day 1 and 2. Not too bad. Of course, I was pretty much out of it. Dave did all the chopping and blending and so on. The blended salad looks like a thick green milkshake. Yuck!

Day 3. Went into kitchen and thought of eating a blended salad for breakfast was too much. Couldn't force myself to do it. Had three pieces of fruit instead. At dinnertime, preparing hot food for the family was very difficult.

Day 4. Managed to eat the blended salad for breakfast. Feel very weak. Had an enormous bowel movement. Couldn't believe I produced it all by myself.

Day 5. Am having constant visions of hot food. I can resign myself to no flesh food, or fish, but oh, for a baked potato or some broccoli with cheese sauce! Or a piece of hot toast with butter on it!

Still feel weak. If I am lying down or sitting down and get up too fast, I get dizzy. Colitis easing up.

Day 6. Christmas Day. How could I penalize my family on this special day? There was a big package of turkey in freezer left over from Thanksgiving. I heated that up, made gravy and candied sweet potatoes, and so on. Then I sat down with my family and slowly drank my green drink — as I have christened my blended salad. The smells and sight of their wonderful food almost drove me mad. When I was doing the dishes I sneaked three bites of turkey and a big spoonful of gravy off one of the plates. This kept me from snapping altogether.

Day 7. Feel weaker than ever. By the time I prepare my food and eat it and clean the juicer and blender, I am done in. I sit down and await next meal time. Am dreaming all the time of hot food. Called Dr. G. He said it was not unusual for people to be weak on this diet. He said, I told you it wouldn't be easy. I can't stand it. I no longer sit at table with family at meals.

Day 9. I cheated today. Bought some bread with no bleaches or preservatives, etc, and toasted a slice, buttered it, and **ATE** it. Closed my eyes while chewing and concentrated on how wonderfully hot it was. Felt much better afterward. Maybe now I can stick to this awful diet a while longer.

Day 10. Not quite as weak. In my memory I relive eating that piece of hot toast. My b.m.'s are getting bigger. Soon I will need a larger toilet bowl. Have lost eight pounds. Went grocery shopping. Bad scene. Never again.

Day 11. I am same as an alcoholic. Can't think of eating this way for a whole month. I keep thinking, one more meal, and then I can bear it.

Still feeling weak. Can't read for very long. Don't usually

watch TV, but find myself watching it for hours. The colitis is gone.

Day 12. Christmas vacation over. Dave went back to work. Stu went back to school. Keith drove back to college. I am alone. Alone with my visions of hot food. Feel like beating my head on the wall. Eating is no fun these days. No comfort or reward either. Just a drag.

Had a friend over for lunch. Prepared tunafish salad for her and ate a very small portion myself. Loved it, but it seemed very salty. I don't feel the least bit guilty about it. Lost ten pounds.

Day 13. Told Dave I **must** have something hot tonight. It won't be meat, it won't have chemicals in it. A baked potato would do it. But he refused to let me. Very easy for him to say so, with a steaming potato on his plate.

Not dizzy anymore. Feel a trifle stronger. Colitis came back briefly. Could it be due to yesterday's tuna?

Day 15. Sneaked some hot food. Again, a piece of unchemicalized bread, toasted, with butter. Closed my eyes and thought of nothing else than the hot crunchy food in my mouth. Divine! But halfway through I was stricken with guilt. Was I undoing the benefits of all those yucky meals.

Day 16. Lost twelve pounds. My clothes hang on me.

Day 18. Felt a head cold coming on yesterday. Ate two whole grapefruit for dinner, nothing else, and went to bed early. No head cold symptoms this morning.

Day 20. Have become accustomed to this rigmarole. Feel well, feel cheerful. Very thirsty for water this week. Returned to work this week.

Am now having a bowel movement after every meal. Big soft ones.

No longer feel like beating my head against the wall.

Day 22. Haven't thought about hot food lately. Someone at work offered me a piece of candy and it was easy to refuse.

When this month is over I don't think I will like salt or sweets anymore.

No bowel movement today. Not surprised. Must be clean as a whistle inside.

Day 23. The weekend. Back to longing for hot food. Also, monotony of this diet is wearing me down. Once again I feel like banging my head on the wall. Have stopped losing weight. Lucky, because I bought some smaller clothing yesterday. My other things hung on me like tents.

Enormous bowel movement this morning after a few sips of my raw vegetable juice. Felt marvelous all day.

Day 24. A work day. Always a little nervous before breakfast. Enormous bowel movement after my juice. What a feeling of well-being follows. Amazing.

Tired by noontime. Don't feel so rebellious about this diet. Maybe because the end is in sight. I'm assuming Dr. G will liberalize it when I see him.

Some celery is more bitter than others. Also cucumbers. Michigan-grown carrots are very bitter. California ones are nicer. Have grown to like the fresh juices and the blended salad but the whole salad without dressing is still no fun.

I think of hot food occasionally, but now it is as if it was something I dimly knew once long ago. No longer think of it with the rampant desire that afflicted me earlier.

Day 25. Bad attack of "I can't believe this happened to me" last night. Cried for hours.

In afternoon, suddenly realized my sinuses have been draining. I can breathe very clearly through my right nostril, and almost so through the other. First time in years!

Called Dr. G. He said the drainage of sinuses is causing my head cold symptoms. Said it is part of the eliminative process and to get more rest. What about work? I asked. Use your own judgment but pace yourself carefully, he replied.

Day 26. Only four more days to go before I see Dr. Goldstein! First day of my menstrual period. Felt tired the last two days, as usual. However, today I don't feel bloated at all, my back doesn't hurt, I am not nervous or irritable, and I have lots of energy.

But what a price I have paid! Eating these yucky foods! Sinuses are partially clogged today, but they are still draining. One small bowel movement today—a mere six inches long. Usually the first day of my period and the day before I am dreadfully constipated.

At day's end, I would say I am having about seventy per cent less discomfort than I generally do the first day of my period. Tummy is, however, slightly swollen.

Day 27. Only three more days! Two bowel movements today. An enormous one before breakfast, and half as much after lunch. My body feels light as a feather.

Day 28. Last night felt very tired after dinner. Got a bad headache, a pain under my left eye. Sinuses clogged, but seem to be draining. Couldn't accomplish any chores around the house.

Today felt tired most of the day. Was glad it was Friday. Tomorrow I see Dr. G for a check up and change in my diet.

Day 29. Saw him. He checked my blood pressure. Asked if any foods disagreed with me. Did not give me any hot foods. Not yet, he said, and changed the subject. Told me to eat one whole papaya every day and add some of its seeds to my blended salad.

Big deal. I was very depressed all day. I had been so hopeful my diet would be liberalized, and my hopes were dashed.

Day 30. Feel very gloomy. Only thing I like about this diet is those big bowel movements. Feel so good after, for hours.

Hid in my den and ate a health food cookie. I used to think they were gummy, but today it tasted wonderful. Nice to eat a different texture of food.

Day 31. No bowel movement today. Could it have been the cookie? Tired soon after dinner. Still depressed because no diet change.

Day 32. Bowel movement this morning, but not as enormous as usual.

Day 34. Enormous b.m. this morning. Even more enormous one late in the evening. That cookie was cooked food, and I guess cooked food contravenes raw food.

Day 35. Have lost much of my yen for hot foods. No b.m. today.

Day 36. Longed for a salami sandwich all day. On pumpernickel bread, mustard on one side, butter on the other, sweet pickles on the side. A favorite since my childhood.

Must have something different to eat. Pineapple! Sent Dave out for one. Tasted great at first — juicy and a crunchy new texture. But soon realized it was downright sour.

Have lost three more pounds. New clothes are getting loose. At work they say I look like a model. Felt very tired from 2:00 PM on.

Day 37. Have been plotting and planning this — this morning got them both out of the house and ate a piece of health bread, toasted and buttered. Sat down with it and didn't read or watch TV or make lists — just closed my eyes and chewed and thought about nothing else.

Didn't taste as great as I remember it.

Day 39. No b.m. for two days. Must have been the toast. When Dr. G says his diet is chemically balanced to be eliminative, he isn't kidding.

Day 40. Once my system got started again, it really started. Three b.m.'s yesterday. I can't believe it.

But do I feel good after each one.

Day 41. Tired spell.

Day 44. Am forgetting about hot food. Because Stuart has been gone all weekend and haven't had to prepare any hot food for him.

Day 46. Feel good. Lots of energy.

Day 47. Beginning to drag.

Day 48. Friday, end of work week. All washed up. Not fit to even sort the laundry. To bed early.

Day 49. Alarmed. Lost more weight. Called Dr. G. He said, don't worry.

Day 50, 51, 52. Bad spell. Pain in right side. Dreadful headache. Dreadful fatigue. Require long naps.

Day 56 and 57. So much work at office! So much pressure! Would like to get out of that job.

Lost another pound. Looked at self in mirror in the nude. My body is so thin it looks child-like. It gave me a very strong feeling of loss. Hipbones like blades, bony bumps on my shoulders, hips flat as a board. Ugh!

Been trying to write an article on the contemporary poet, Sylvia Plath. A literary mag editor wants it. May never get up enough energy to do it. Tired, tired. Something has got to go. The writing, I suppose. But it is so dear to my heart.

Day 58. Saturday. Five hours overtime today. Tired, tired.

Day 60. Had a b.m. that must have been at least two feet long. That literary mag woman wants me on her editorial board. Such a compliment! I will try.

Day 66. Colitis is back with a bang. Constant pain, lots of gas, and the gas is stuck inside me. No diarrhea, though.

Day 72. Dr. G said I could have have cooked vegetables. Had this wonderful baked potato.

Day 73. Slept all weekend. Gave up the raw salad. Colitis easing up. Been snarling at my family. Even Stuart catches it. I used to worry so about hurting other's feelings — not any more. Now I feel like riding roughshod over anybody who gets in my way. It is as if my body is so absorbed with saving itself there's nothing left for being nice to people. Can't plan ahead; made an engagement to go shopping with a girl friend from work, but when it came time to go, I simply couldn't.

Day 79. Colitis has eased up some. Have had short spells of feeling cheerful and optimistic. Dr. G says I **must** have more rest. Ha! I have a new supervisor, a man who used to run the department in the past. They say he is power-mad. Working with him isn't going to be any fun.

CHAPTER IV

Colitis and Other Problems

As I have mentioned, my colitis gave me many problems with the diet. If a person has a condition which is soothed by cooked, bland, smooth foods, you can easily imagine what is going to happen when most everything you put in your mouth is **RAW**. Eventually I became accustomed to the raw vegetable juices and the raw blended salad and they tasted okay. The raw nuts, however, gave me an ongoing problem, and at times I would not eat them, focusing on the raw milk unsalted cheddar cheese.

Dr. G suggested I chop the nuts, soak overnight in the refrigerator in apple juice. Then the next day, whiz in blender and eat with spoon. I tried it once, with peanuts, but it didn't work. It was a lot of extra work and the end result was about as appetizing as baby food.

My nerves were very bad and I kept badgering him until he let me take some B vitamins. He suggested a certain brand, which he knew was made in the best possible manner. I tried them and they helped a great deal.

I'm sure you can imagine how boring the diet was. Also, at times I felt like a rabbit. Dining out in restaurants was, of course, a forbidden pleasure. Not that my doctor forbade it, but how could I observe my diet when everything served in restaurants is cooked, salted, and made from foods loaded with additives? Dave, of course, often lunched in restaurants with friends from work and he could eat anything he wanted.

It was an entire year before we could eat out together. Dr. G had just made the Grand Announcement that I could eat fish. So we went to a restaurant which broiled fresh-caught fish and cooked fresh (not canned) vegetables. This place serves large portions. The fish tasted heavenly, and I ate every bite.

About one hour later that unaccustomed load of food hit me. It hit me so hard I had to go straight to bed. I could feel that big meal stuck just below my sternum. It gave me a very uncomfortable night's sleep, and I couldn't get out of bed till about noon the next day. It was a very unhappy ending and put a finish to restaurant eating for me for quite a while.

Most of our lives we had too many other obligations to be able to afford travel. Earlier, back in 1977, Dave decided he wanted to revisit the places in Europe where he had served in the Army during World War II, and so we took a trip there. Dave learned that he loved to travel, and in September, 1979, decided he wanted to return to Europe. If I went with him, it would mean a great deal of restaurant eating. I wasn't too keen on it, but he wanted me along for company. Dave argued that perhaps in Europe they did not process and adulterate their food as much. Dr. G gave a reluctant blessing; do the best you can, he said; you've had almost two years of good diet, it may protect you. Just don't eat meat.

So we went abroad and toured in six different countries. We rented a car and traveled without previously made hotel reservations. This meant every day around 4:00 PM we had to begin looking for a place to stay. Dave thrived on this; to him, it meant adventure. To me, it meant nervous tension. Not knowing where I was going to put my head down at night was nerve-racking. Also, a satisfactory room did not always appear on cue. There was a lot of looking for a place, getting out and inquiring as to availability and price, and then looking at the room to see if it was clean and if the bed was firm. And if not, getting back in the car and looking for another place.

My stomach felt uncomfortable with all the heavy, cooked food and I became dreadfully constipated. Toward the end of our trip, that was all I could think about. Not even suppositories would work. Raw fruit was hard to find and salads as we know them were non-existent. Apparently the climate does not permit the growing of head lettuce and other greens. When you asked for "salat" you usually received cooked sliced potatoes, beets, carrots, served cold, lying on one limp leaf of pale green lettuce.

Dave was very pleased with the trip, but then he was a healthy person on an ordinary diet. I, too, could have enjoyed the scenic beauties and grand old buildings if I weren't afraid I was poisoning myself with every mouthful of food.

When we came back home the first thing I did was take a coffee enema. Dr. G did not approve of this — he said enemas take minerals out of the system — but I was so uncomfortable I had to. My raw diet kept my b.m.'s moving briskly and as a result when I was constipated I was extremely uncomfortable.

I had heard about coffee enemas at the Cancer Seminar I'd attended, which I mentioned in Chapter Two. The coffee goes promptly through the walls of the intestines to the liver, which, recognizing it as a poison, is stimulated to work quickly to throw it off, and along with it, other poisons that are in the system.

I took these enemas two days in a row. I found that they did not make me feel shivery and quaky, as other enemas did in the past. In comparison, they were almost soothing. After the second one I felt immensely better. The caffeine gave me an energy charge for the rest of the day, and my goodness, how nice to feel energetic for a change, instead of all dragged out.

However, with resumption of my raw diet, my old friend, colitis, kicked in and for a few days I had to go on an all bland diet — oatmeal, soft boiled eggs, cream soups.

In January of 1980 public television ran a 2.5 hour story on Joan Robinson, who, when dying of cancer, had allowed cameras to enter her home. The whole town was talking about this show, and it had gotten lots of coverage in the daily papers. I didn't want to watch it, but I was drawn to it like a moth to the flame.

Mrs. Robinson went the conventional medical route; they operated and operated, about a dozen times or more. She was wearing a colostomy bag on the outside and her rate of excretion kept slowing down. Her doctors wished to perform another operation but she was so weak the anesthetist refused to administer anesthesia one more time. Mrs. Robinson, of course, died.

I couldn't get over the way those doctors cut and cut into that poor woman, and how much pain she suffered, and they didn't stop until her body would not take another operation.

I knew, then, THAT I HAD CHOSEN THE RIGHT COURSE. I might be nervous, and I might get terribly tired, but I was functioning, I was taking care of my house, and my body was whole. But I couldn't forget Mrs. Robinson. I was haunted by that familiar saying, There but for the grace of God, go I. In my case, it was, There but for the grace of Dr. Goldstein, go I. I felt like the ghost at the feast.

Sleepless nights followed. Tensions mounted. It was a very cold month and when I went out into the cold, severe fatigue set in.

I began feeling many pains in my breasts. It settled down to a persistent ache deep in my right breast. It became painful to move my arm. This was the start of a new lump, I knew from past experience. Was I that much better off than the lady on television who died? It seemed every other article I picked up was yammering about the quality of life . . . ha! There was no redeeming quality to the life I was leading.

I hated to call Dr. Goldstein again. I knew his time was valuable, and I had not needed an office visit for a long time. He might resent my being such a pest. Often I would study my book on herb remedies rather than bother him. But this was really serious. I called and he listened to my story and he asked if I had pain in the armpits. I said no.

He suggested I apply mild, moist heat to my breast for twenty minutes, three times a day. Also, to eat only raw foods for three days. Nothing cooked. Eat protein twice during the day. No starches in the evening. I followed his suggestions.

The results were good. The pain and the ache went away. Once again, my immune system had rescued me, all by itself, thanks to the fact I had corrected my diet. Once again, Dr. Goldstein had proved himself a genius in my eyes.

When I first discovered my cancer, back in 1977, that was about the time there was so much publicity in the papers about hair dye causing cancer. The dye manufacturers put up a big howl, but the FDA was adamant. Eventually the manufacturers changed their formulations and supposedly . . . hopefully . . . the dye was no longer cancer-causing.

I, of course, had stopped dying my hair as soon as Dr. G had advised against putting chemicals into my system. My hair had started to turn gray soon after my first son was born. As a baby, he was fussy and screamed a lot. That didn't fit in with my concept of what babies were like, and caused me a lot of distress. I used to make jokes that when the Stork brought my first baby, he also brought my first gray hairs.

About the time that hair dye came under scrutiny, that was about the time that dozens of things were written up as cancer-causing, from artificial sugar to nitrates to industrial pollutants. So many things came under fire that it got to be a joke. Journalists fashioned entire columns about it, saying it was almost too dangerous to live. They were using humor to mask fear, and I can understand this ploy. If we can laugh about something unpleasant, it's easier to handle.

Dave and I were just as uneasy as anyone else, and this constant barrage of articles about cancer-causing things in our food and environment led us to begin a general study of this entire grisly topic.

The Detroit Chapter of Foundation for Alternative Cancer Therapies (FACT) was, during 1978, sponsoring informational meetings one night a month, and they were an excellent source of information of the kind one would never get from ordinary sources.

The problem with attending them was the timing. These meetings were held in evenings. I was tired from working all day, and it was the dead of winter. Going out into the frigid weather added to my fatigue. Dave would drive me, and I would bring pen and paper so I could take notes. Quite often the approach was so new to my mind that I couldn't understand it. At one time I would have thought, how dare they question our heroic doctors? What a bunch of quacks! But now it was different. I myself was using an alternative therapy.

At one of the meetings the speaker encouraged cancer patients in the audience to stand up and own up to their condition and state their therapy. I stood up, too, and with a great quivering of my knees, stated my condition out loud.

After the meeting a woman came up to me and we began talking. She had cancer that was spreading to her lungs and was interested in taking an alternative method, but was scared to. She had a lot of confidence in her doctor, and she wasn't sure an alternative would do the trick. Her husband, on the other hand, felt that conventional treatment was not helping his wife, and he'd investigated and decided that Dr. Rheem's method was better. I have not been able to locate a written statement of Dr. Rheem's method; so I am not sure that what I say is accurate; in fact, I am not 100 per cent sure of the spelling of his name.

However, from what I recall, it was a very vigorous therapy involving a complete change in diet and preparing large quantities of distilled water mixed with fresh lemon juice and drinking a certain number of ounces every two hours, throughout the day, even during the night. Her husband, in order to encourage her to try this method, had gone on it himself, since he had various ailments which it probably would help.

People at the office teased him about the jug of water on his desk, but he ignored them. As time went by he began feeling better and his ailments cleared up.

We arranged for this couple to come to our house for a visit. With them they brought a very helpful book, RAW VEGETABLE JUICES, by Dr. N. W. Walker, which they left with me.

An interesting thing she told me was that after a previous operation to remove cancerous growth she'd been told to go in weekly for radiation. She did so and the treatments laid her low. She tried to find out from the X-ray technician how long she would have to continue, but he was evasive. Later on she insisted on knowing, and was told that perhaps she didn't really need it, but she was part of a control group. She found this callous and frightening, and stopped going. It made her wonder how much of what doctors do for cancer patients is merely experimental, but is presented as if it is the proven thing.

This lady did go on Dr. Rheem's regimen for a few months, but then panicked and submitted to another operation. She later died.

I began studying Dr. Walker's little book. Upon my first reading I was put off somewhat by the tone of the book. In my opinion it seemed strident, almost fanatic. But I was amazed to notice the book had first been published in 1936 and the copy I held in my hand, back then in 1978, was the 27th Edition, Revised and Enlarged. The book explains, with much scientific detail, what raw juices are, why they are good for you, and gives formulas for juice combinations for every possible ailment.

Dr. Walker says that most cancer patients are stuffed full of resentment and until they get rid of it, they will never get rid of their cancer. I had a big problem accepting this statement and in applying it to myself. I was not aware of feeling resentful. I was aware of feeling depressed and angry, but not resentful. I had many other things to worry about then, so I gave up trying to figure out this fine point. Now I realize that resentment is just another side of a many-sided coin bearing the names anger, depression, hostility, bitterness, desire for revenge, and God alone knows what other negative emotion.

I also realize now (in 1987) that Dr. Walker's book is the kind of book that takes repeated reading over a period of time. As I look it over now, it seems quite clear. I believe it is because in the intervening ten years I have gained much background information that enables me to understand it fully in a manner that was not possible when I was not in the habit of thinking deeply or carefully about health information.

Laetrile came into the news and it was frequently appearing in the headlines. Doctors regularly said there was no evidence that it was useful. Yet in 1978 I knew a man who had advanced cancer, was a dreadful yellow color, and could not eat. He went to Mexico and received Laetrile and several months later was eating, going to work, and had a normal color.

I came across a book, LAETRILE CASE HISTORIES by John A. Richardson, M.D., and Patricia Griffin, R.N. This book tells Dr. Richardson's story. He was a California physician who gave Laetrile to hopeless cancer patients and saw them recover. When the California branch of the American

Medical Association discovered what he was doing, he was hounded out of practice in a thoroughly brutal manner.

In this book he reveals a very pertinent reason why Laetrile will never be accepted by the medical establishment. Laetrile (also called amygdalin) is B-17, which is a vitamin, which is a food stuff, and as such is not patentable.

What does this mean?

It means there is no fortune in it for the drug companies, and no fees for doctors for writing prescriptions.

Another thing I have been told is that new doctors are sometimes started out in practice by low-interest loans from drug companies, in return for prescribing that firm's products and some doctors quite often get kickbacks from pharmacists. Also, doctors quite often own pharmacies. To me, this shows there is a vested interest in prescribing drugs rather than change in diet as a treatment for cancer.

I did not "enjoy" reading Dr. Richardson's book. There were too many harsh truths in it. But I learned to think in terms of the money angle—that is to say, what groups have an interest in keeping things the way they are.

CHAPTER V

Trying to Understand Cancer

Dave and I continued our studies. It gradually dawned on us that Dr. Goldstein was not the only doctor who had devised an alternative cancer therapy. Several others had— Dr. Kelley, Dr. Gerson, Dr. Rheems, Dr. Wigmore, Dr. Contreras, and Dr. Manner. While not arriving there via the same path, they shared a common goal—to avoid the conventional methods of radiation and chemotherapy which were so depleting and harmful to the body. And there was one thing in common—they all involved a drastic change in eating habits.

I managed to obtain a photocopy of the diet recommended by Dr. Contreras of Tijuana, Mexico, which he uses in conjunction with enemas and Laetrile. When I saw it, I was amazed. It was similar to Dr. Goldstein's in many ways—no meat, no white flour, no white sugar, no canned food, no processed food.

A pamphlet put out by the Foundation for Alternative Cancer Therapies (FACT), from the headquarters in New York City, says, "CANCER IS NOT THE TUMOR." This is where conventional medicine makes its big mistake. They attack the tumor. They bombard it with big guns.

But the tumor is the net result of things going wrong in the body. A person's metabolic balance is thrown off kilter by wrong eating and/or lots of stress and/or exposure to carcinogens in the environment or the work place. The immune system breaks down and cancer is allowed to start.

I went to a speech given by Dr. Harold Manner, head of the Biology Department at Loyola University and he said something very disturbing. He is one of the doctors mentioned above with a new therapy. He said that everyone gets cancer about once a week because our foods are so highly processed and adulterated and our environment so polluted. He also said everyone has a built-in protector—the immune system, which destroys cancer cells.

Dr. Manner's therapy involves change in diet, emulsified vitamins, and Laetrile. I believe he also uses enemas. The Laetrile is given only at a certain point in the therapy. Dr. Manner has since retired.

Let's consider the things listed above that cause cancer. Can you change the air? Can you change your work place? Can you avoid all stress? Not very easily. But can you change your eating habits? Yes, it is possible.

That's what I did, and what was the cost? It cost $140 for a juicer, $80 for a heavy duty blender, and $20 a week for vegetables. (We have saved thousands on the meat bill.) In 1984, they said it costs the average cancer patient $30,000 to die. I heard of one case when it cost over $100,000. Where does this money go? It is divided up between doctors, hospitals, and drug companies.

However, changing one's eating habits is not easy. I think it's because food is not merely food to most of us. It is a tranquilizing act, feeding yourself; that's why airlines are always feeding you in flight, to keep your anxiety down. Food is also a pleasure, just from the taste of good things. It is a pleasure from the socializing aspect because it's so nice dining with friends. It is a comfort when things go wrong. It is a reward after a long hard day at work. It is a punishment when something pricks our conscience. When you've broken your reducing diet, food soothes you and punishes you both at the same time. All in all, eating is a complex activity.

Sweets, in particular, remind you of pleasurable childhood experiences when your daddy or mommy gave you a sucker, or bought you an ice cream cone, or put a birthday cake in front of you. That sweet dependency of childhood is a delightful state we all want to go back to now and then, and what better way than to eat foods given you in those luminous days of childhood.

I saw a little saying on a calendar once, and I don't recall it exactly, but it went something like this, "I wish I were a child again, colors have never been so bright since then."

That saying is so true! I can still remember the taste of the first ice cream cone I ever had. It was at the Great Lakes Exhibition in Cleveland, Ohio, and I was about nine years of age. My father took me there to see all the wonderful sights. He bought me a cone. It was filled with orange sherbet, and I was surprised and thrilled by the new taste, color and texture. If I live to be a hundred, I will never again eat orange sherbet that tastes as wonderful as it did the first time I ever ate it. It is tied in with memories of my father, whom I adored and whom I only saw once a week.

With all these complexities and meanings attached to food, changing one's eating habits involves a great deal of self-discipline and self-denial. A certain friend asked for my diet for reducing purposes (Lord, does it reduce you! First you gradually get skinny, you stay that way about six months, and then you gradually return to a normal weight) and I gave it to her. She couldn't stay on the diet for two days. Some people can't deny themselves anything. To be sure, it is hard to give up everything you are accustomed to and all your favorites. When you have to learn strange new ways of preparing food. When these new ways consume far more time than you usually give to food preparing. It can be done, but it isn't easy. A person has to be seriously motivated.

It was lucky that Dave and I continued our studies, for the more we understood, the stronger my motivation for sticking to the diet, and the stronger was Dave's motivation for seeing that I did. Because, as I mentioned earlier in my diary, there were times when I felt like I would beat my head against the wall if I didn't have something hot or something different. I'd say, I'm going to have a hot dog, just one, and he'd say, No, you're not. Then I'd say, I'm going to have a bagel, and he'd say, No, you're not.

As we studied, we learned that the work of Dr. Ernest Krebs was responsible for enabling doctors to conceive the metabolic approach to cancer. The way Dr. Krebs worked it out is very technical and I will not attempt to reproduce it here. What shocked me was that he arrived at his thesis in the early 1900's. And it has been almost entirely ignored.

I have often wondered why the medical establishment, aside from the profit motive, is so hostile to his theory. I have come across one partial explanation. It came about accidentally while I was researching an historical novel I was writing. The novel was taking place in England in 1816 and the action was such that I needed to know what was going on in medicine at that time. While we were in London in 1980 I read a lot of old medical books written during the early 1800's. It appears that in Europe the basic approach has always been to be cautious, to wait and see, perhaps to change the patient's habits and attitudes. They felt that patients eventually got better, regardless of how much medication they took or what the doctor did to them. Another strong thread was the concept that the patient's own personality was responsible both for the illness and the type of illness.

In America, in the early 1800's, a different philosophy was developing, one of BIG HEROICS. No "wait and see." Rather, it was, let the treatment be drastic; let's give strong medicine and lots of it. Let us always intervene. Let us operate and the sooner the better. This approach to illness would naturally lead to the idea of attacking cancer with big guns, scuttling the possibility that correcting the chemical balance within the body might be helpful.

With this sort of background, when President Nixon declared a "War on Cancer" in the early 1970's the public and doctors were ready and waiting. Declaring "war" summons up military comparisons, to which the public is accustomed, and makes it easy to come up with catchy slogans.

In my opinion, this war on cancer was one of the worst things that ever happened. It began with a modest budget of a few million, now it's in the hundreds of millions. According to a publication of the American Cancer Society, dated 1984, which I have in my hands at this very moment, they disbursed $231,200,000 in funds. That is not chicken feed.

This publication also provides a summary of research grants and fellowships they awarded during fiscal year ended August 31, 1983. The total amount was $56,632,563. It was disbursed to 151 research facilities.

Many hospitals have huge research wings devoted to seeking out causes and treatments. These wings are full of scientists and technicians busily doing experiments, peering into microscopes and writing memos to each other.

President Nixon's War on Cancer no doubt sprang from a wish to help people but it has spawned a monster.

Cancer is now a multi-million dollar industry, and who wants to cut off the funds by finding the cause or the cure? Who wants to throw all these people out of work? It is better for them to say, "Gee whiz! There are dozens of different kinds of cancer, and each one has a different cause, it's going to take a long time!"

This is a slick dodge. As it appears to me, after my years of study, that while cancer assumes many forms, there is only one underlying cause for cancer — an imbalance of the body's chemistry which throws the immune system out of balance.

The immune system is part of the defense system of the

body. It is like the White Knight who comes charging to the rescue. Doctors don't know a lot about it, because it is very complex and difficult to keep track of during experiments. But they do know that when it detects something harmful to the body (bacteria, viruses, drugs, pollens, insect venoms, chemicals, foods, foreign tissue, and cancerous cells) it forms an antibody specific for the harmful thing which is to be attacked.

When the body's immune system is low, due to a variety of possible causes, then illness can strike.

Throughout our studies, every now and then I'd wonder what I had done to bring on my cancer. I wanted to pin it down, neatly and conclusively, on **one** causative factor. For a period of five years, ages 29 to 34, I'd taken the contraceptive pill. Earlier, ages 26 and 27, I'd taken monthly hormone shots to ease severe bouts of premenstrual tension.

When I reached my forties I had a friend who was a "health nut" and under her influence I reduced the amount of beef and junk food I ate.

When, at 49, I suddenly got cancer, I thought it must go back to the earlier years when I'd put hormones into my system. When I expressed these thoughts to Dr. Goldstein's wife, Corinne, who is a very knowledgeable lady, she said perhaps it was also the severe stress I'd been enduring for the five years just prior.

I must tell you a little about Corinne, she is a fabulous person. When her husband went on his raw vegetable diet, she put herself and her sons on the same diet. When I met her I was stunned by the beauty of her hair and skin. Such glossy hair and smooth skin! And she was so ideally slender! When I asked her what she did for her skin and hair, she said, "Nothing, I just eat right."

To return to the issue of stress. My tensions began with my second marriage and increased when I transferred to a job in a new field, then tripled when I got a new supervisor. There was more stress when I learned of my cancer and my family began reacting to this unhappy news. But at the time I didn't realize all this was stress — I thought it was just daily life.

I kept thinking about Corinne's remark that stress may cause cancer. I mentioned it to Dr. Goldstein, and he said "Yes, stress is the ultimate cause of disease." I simply could not understand this. For one thing, I never had any scientific training and it was hard to interpret this new information. High school chemistry had been one of the most traumatic experiences in my life. I worked like a dog to get a "C" and I suspect I got it only because the teacher knew how hard I tried.

For another reason, the entire slant of the medical profession, as it trickles down to the layman, is that disease is caused by something from **outside the body** — bacteria, or viruses, or as we say in common parlance during our North American winters, the flu bug's got me.

Since I'd spent almost fifty years with this mind slant, it was hard to change over. I was beginning to understand metabolic therapy and the role of the immune system, but to take it a step further and understand that stress caused cancer was just too much for me at the time. I said to myself, Dr. G is a brilliant chemist, and I must continue to trust him.

I believe it was during 1980 that I was driving in my car and a local talk show hostess began reading a newly released report. A doctor had put together a personality profile of a person likely to get heart disease. He called it Type "A" personality. The various traits were listed and the fact that this personality type was a certain per cent more likely to get heart disease. The hostess went on to say that when these Type A's reacted in their typical ways, they were putting lots of stress on themselves. Yes, I thought, I can see that. Then she went on to say these Type A's were also prone to get certain other diseases, one of which was cancer. When she said this, I almost drove off the road.

I tried to think back to the traits she'd mentioned, and they seemed to apply more to ambitious businessmen than to myself. So I temporarily shelved the whole concept of stress causing disease in the back of my mind.

In 1980 my cancer seemed to be laying low. My body was not developing any new lumps. My nerves were a little better. But I was lonely staying at home. Vera, my mother-in-law, was home with me, of course, but she was very quiet and not much company. I went through a long spell of missing work and my "sisters" back there, and the companionship of other people in general; I even missed the routine. I thought about getting a part-time job. The only place that was interested in women of my age was K-Mart, the discount department store, and I knew that standing on hard floors all day would hurt my feet too much.

One day while I was home a volunteer came to the door and asked for a donation to the American Cancer Society. I looked at her, aghast. Give to the American Cancer Society? To the outfit that seemed to be in the business of perpetuating cancer, not eradicating it? I couldn't give money to a group I didn't believe in. I fumbled mentally to find an excuse, and ended up telling her my husband contributed at the office. After I shut the door, I leaned against it as emotions swirled through me so strongly I could have fallen over.

Chicken, I sneered to myself. Too chicken to tell her you wouldn't contribute because you believe cancer research is on the wrong track. You've always been chicken when it comes to facing up to other people. In fact, most of your life you've been too chicken to even have your own opinion.

When you were young, society said get married and have kids. You wanted to be a novelist; did you ever say, "Listen, world, I want to be different. Kids might take up all my time and energy and nothing will be left for creating, maybe I should go my own way." Did you? Not you, you weak-spined little mouse.

Joyce Carol Oates said that to herself. She married, but she made a conscious decision not to have kids, and look at her now. About fifteen books published, she grinds one out every year; her stories get chosen for the annual book, Best Short Stories of the Year, even Time magazine writes about her. And who has heard about you? Nobody.

Too stupid to think for yourself. Too weak to stand up for yourself. If you had stood up to Mr. Hamm right in the beginning, I bet he'd have treated you differently. Your co-worker held her own and he treats her differently. You are a wimp.

But you did one thing right. When they said, let's cut off your breast, you said, "No." You went your own way. Maybe there is hope for you, after all.

CHAPTER VI

Panic Strikes Again

In April of 1980 I received a brochure telling about a big writer's conference to be held at Indiana University the following June. It was to last a week. I was very interested in attending because they were having four big-time editors and agents from New York. And — best of all — these big-shots had promised to READ all manuscripts submitted during the course of the conference. I had never even seen an editor from New York in person; my only contact had been via submissions sent through the mail. What a chance!

Classes and workshops both were offered. The workshops were being taught by big-name authors with many credits. Any prospective student could attend classes, but he could not attend workshops unless he was accepted beforehand. To do this the student had to submit a manuscript well before the conference. A certain level of professional ability had to be displayed in his MS or he would not be accepted.

I decided to try for both fiction and poetry workshops. I sent in the first ten pages of the detective novel I was working on, and six of my poems, and sat back to wait. When I received Indiana University's letter of acceptance, my joy knew no bounds. I was so happy I practically went into orbit. Then, about a week later, I had a new lump in my breast.

I called Dr. G and told him about it, saying nothing unusually stressful had happened and I couldn't understand it. He questioned me a bit and I revealed how happy I'd been about my acceptance to the workshops. He said **that** was probably the cause, that **positive stress** — i.e., excessive joy — could also cause lumps.

I asked him whether I should continue with my plans to go to the conference. I was almost locked into it; I had sent my money in and it was beyond the refund date. He suggested that I go, taking my diet with me.

At first I thought, how is it possible? But I did it.

I took enough distilled water to last the entire week. I took my blender, a big head of romaine lettuce, a large sack of apples, a large sack of oranges, and plenty of notepaper and three pens.

How to get there was the next problem. No planes and no trains went to Bloomington, Indiana, and my stamina was too low to permit me to drive myself there. In the end Dave drove me and left the car with me. A friend who was visiting relatives nearby came and picked him up. This meant I would somehow have to drive myself home. I planned to leave early and drive home in easy stages.

As we drove there, I wondered how to explain my diet to my roommate. Alas, it turned out my roommate was the wife of a doctor. With that in her background, I knew her mind would be closed to the idea that diet could cure cancer. But I explained it the best I could, not mentioning my cancer, rather using my colitis as an excuse. She was very polite about it, but I could tell she thought I was nutty as a fruitcake.

One piece of luck, though, there was a refrigerator in our room, and I could put my food supplies in there.

Indiana University has a lovely campus and the building where we were housed, the Student Union, was built in a classical style and looked brand new. The interior was in perfect condition. After a few days, however, I noticed that the trees and shrubbery beds surrounding the building were very mature. Upon inquiry, I learned it was about twenty years old. I couldn't believe it. There wasn't one sign of student damage anywhere.

There was another stroke of luck awaiting me. Right in the same building were a cafeteria and several restaurants. One was a hamburger place, one was a health food restaurant, and the cafeteria served many meatless dishes. The health food restaurant offered an enormous salad bar. There were so many items that you put your paper plate on a scale and you paid according to how much it weighed.

I was in seventh heaven. I ate an apple and orange at breakfast and made my green drink once in the morning, then ate in the restaurants for the other meals. Most evenings, I indulged in one dish of hot food, usually a vegetable and cheese casserole.

I was too busy to pay attention to my body, but sometime near the end of the week I checked and discovered that the lump had disappeared. A miracle, of my own body, by its immune system, without the big guns of chemotherapy or radiation or surgery. I've looked up my notes and it took four weeks to get rid of the lump.

Readers may ask, how did I know when these recurring lumps were cancerous? This was a question that bothered me. Dave would sometimes say, You are getting all upset over nothing, it may be an ordinary lump. I did some careful study and self-observation and concluded as follows: a cancerous lump is very hard; it does not move easily; it usually gives pain.

In contrast, a benign lump is soft and freely movable and doesn't cause pain.

The general scenario that precedes getting a bad lump is like this . . . first, a feeling of soreness, then tension and tightness, which may go on for a while; then the lump. The pain may come with the lump, or after it, or just before it.

Let me tell you about the kinds of pain. Sometimes it's like needles, short and stabbing; sometimes like tearing ripsaws; or like hard-edged jabs of lightning. The fright they bring with them is as bad as the pain itself. A host of visions grab you. Will you lose your independence because you can't care for yourself? Will you then be dependent on the good will of others? What a stinging loss of pride this brings. It's bad at any age, but in middle age it is humbling, humiliating.

You wonder, how severe will this pain be, the one I'm having now? Sometimes my breasts were so full of pain that I couldn't clench my hands to pick things up. How long will this pain last? Will you be able to walk when it is over? If it proves to be a short-lived pain, you are thankful. You can still move about, you can still do for yourself.

Another thing I suffered was mixed feelings about my sexuality. I was somehow disgusted with that part of myself. I felt tainted. It is hard to be interested in love-making when you feel that way. When I went through the motions, hoping for some response inside me, it wasn't really me lying there in the bed, it was some big wax doll who looked like me but had sawdust inside.

Despite my feelings I never denied Dave very often. I knew how important it was to him. I remembered how enthusiastic I used to be about love-making and it was like a fading dream I had in another life. But since it was important to Dave, I did my best to oblige him.

1980 was a watershed year. It was the last year that my older son, Keith, was home. He'd be away for a while, then he'd come home. He and Dave were, it seemed, locked in a battle to the death. That year I discovered lumps in my breast, one or both, on three different occasions. I had severe bouts of flu, head colds, and a bladder infection. These illnesses hung on. Keith's behavior became more and more bizarre.

At times my colitis was so severe I couldn't eat. This would lead to being too hungry to sleep. Since I couldn't take sleeping pills, insomnia came to be a way of life. I went around with a constant pain in my abdomen and in my mind. What is worth living about this? I wondered. The first year I was sick, I fought the idea of dying; it terrified me; but during 1980 there were times when death seemed a pleasant alternative.

Two or three times I fell off my diet with a big bang. I couldn't help it; my colitis would be so severe my system could not digest raw food. When I fell off and ate bland, cooked foods, I would get dreadfully constipated; but at least the pain in my intestines eased off. I was very careful not to tell Dr. Goldstein when I had fallen off. Not that he would have scolded me; he understands people are only human. But I didn't want him to think less of me.

It was becoming very apparent that my returning health was not returning in any steady upward line. It was not even resting on any plateaus. I would feel better for a few hours, or half a day, then my energy nosedived and I could barely drag myself through the house.

Dave read an article saying that people who didn't eat meat often needed iron. I began taking an all-day iron capsule made from yeast. There was an improvement in my energy level right away. Not as much as I would have wished, but certainly better.

One mood that was very prevalent in me during some of these years was one of frustration over my lack of energy, my inability to participate in all the activities I was accustomed to doing, in terms of personal life and household management. It was hard enough to do the very basic routines of life . . . getting up, taking a shower, brushing my teeth, scrubbing vegetables, preparing them, eating them. I learned that I had to eat sitting down, also to eat slowly, and this took up precious time. Sometimes the raw food would hit my system hard, and the very act of digestion wore me down.

To alleviate the symptoms of my colitis, I had to develop a new approach to eating. No more eating on the run, no more grabbing a quick bite. As mentioned in the previous paragraph, I learned I had to eat slowly. Dr. G often mentioned his diet had to be eaten slowly, to allow digestion to begin in the mouth. The next thing was to avoid all unpleasantness at the table. No family squabbles. No violence on television. I would have been much happier to have the television off during dinner, but Dave had the habit of watching the evening sports. A certain local sportscaster was a great favorite of his. I gave in on this point; it was either that, or have meals ready earlier. But Vera liked to eat at a certain time, and I felt the poor old lady had already given up so much, at least she could have her meals when she wanted them.

The next thing was, upon finishing my meal, not to jump right up and start the dishes, which had been a necessary habit during all those years I worked. Not to jump up, not to read, not to watch television, just to sit quietly. This habit of sitting quietly for five minutes proved to be very beneficial. Then, when I got up from the table, it was important not to rush into washing the dishes quickly so I could rush into the next chore. Rather, to go into it slowly—without a sense of rushing through it.

Let me tell you, it took a lot of work on myself to get rid of the habit of rushing through my activities. I still don't have my new habit firmly in place, and I am compelled to wonder why good habits are so hard to form.

I have tried many different mental tricks to get my body rid of its rush-rush habits. One of them was something I'd heard about Buddhist monks, that they tried to perform each action slowly and gracefully and beautifully, whether it was pouring a cup of tea or hoeing in the garden, their thoughts involved only in the action itself. This certainly was what I needed. I observed that my thoughts were often running ahead of what I was doing, to the next chore, and the one after that, to thoughts of how many I had to do, how little time I had, and how little energy.

And, of course, there was another acute source of frustration, my not having enough energy to pursue my writing. This particular frustration had been a constant one for years. And, as I've mentioned, it was one that caused me deep unhappiness. I think God meant me to be a writer; why else does the yearning never leave me? I do wish He wouldn't put so many obstacles in my way.

When I was at work, it appeared that I was the only one in my division who suffered from colitis. Ulcers seemed to be the common problem, plus several people had hemorrhoids. As time has gone by, however, I realize colitis is fairly common, at least in middle-aged people. It seems most of us are born healthy, and it takes years of improper eating, impure food, and constant rush-rush to take their toll.

I think working for big companies is very stressful. I grant you that working for a living itself is plenty stressful these days, no matter where, but I think there is an extra dimension when the company is large. It makes you feel like a number. Company policies must be followed, or nothing would get done, but after a time this becomes dehumanizing. Everyone wants to feel unique and important and appreciated in the work place, and while you may get this in a small company (if management is humane) you are almost certain not to find it in a big firm.

When I first went to work for X Mfg. Company, I was very reluctant to do so because of its bigness. However, it was 1970 and America was "enjoying" one of its recessions and I could find nothing else. Actually, I fell into my job accidentally. I had signed up to work for a temporary service, and they sent me to X Mfg. for three weeks, to substitute for a secretary who needed a leg operation.

It turned out that the assignment was in the export finance department and since they dealt with Latin America I had to type letters in Spanish. In college I'd had two years of Spanish and it came back to me, enough so that I could type the letters quite rapidly. My boss, Mr. Cowl, was so pleased with my performance that he insisted I go to Division Personnel and fill out an application before I left. I demurred, saying there were no openings. But he insisted, and I complied.

Lo and behold, three weeks later I was called in for an interview by the Marketing Department. Here again my Spanish abilities were a plus. I was told that if I would refresh my Spanish at night school, I would be hired, and they would pay for my tuition. That was an offer I couldn't refuse, so I agreed.

When I first began to work there, I soon noticed that many of the men, especially those of middle-age stuck in dead-end jobs, seemed very resentful of the company, as if it were a nasty rigid father figure ready to spank them at every turn. These men often were downright hostile. I thought, how sad, how wasteful, I'm never going to waste my emotions that way. Alas, two years later I was showing signs of the same resentment and hostility toward management. It must be something in the air, like a flu bug you can't escape.

My first boss was Mr. Holly. I worked for him for one year, then my job as his secretary was eliminated and I was transferred to the Parts Department. A new product was being taken on and a new price list was needed, and overtime was granted. Most of the women refused overtime; they were making good money and the overtime put them into a higher tax bracket and the extra money they netted was not worth the extra fatigue.

I, however, being a new employee, was not making all that much and I netted more from overtime. I was asked to work on the new parts price list and I accepted. It was not secretarial work, but clerical work involving calculating and proofreading. It was a little tricky becoming familiar with the part numbers, which were lengthy combinations of letters and numbers.

The supervisor for this project was Dave Greenfield and

we worked closely together. I had been divorced six years. Dave and his wife had had a platonic marriage for many years, with a "gentleman's agreement" between them that they would stay together until their children finished high school. I came into Dave's life at this point and our association grew into something more. After a year-long courtship we decided to marry.

During our courtship we had kept our dating secret from other people in the office. When an office romance is common knowledge and then it fizzles, it is very embarrassing for the parties concerned. Also, the bosses don't like it because they feel too much time gets wasted as the parties visit back and forth.

We planned a simple ceremony, but it was very difficult making the arrangements during working hours. I couldn't use the phone on my desk without being overheard, so I went down to the lobby during my break to use the pay phone. I felt like a sneak; if someone saw me they would wonder what I was up to. Quite often I had to wait around for the phones to be free; they were often tied up by salesmen checking in with their offices. But I did manage to arrange for the cake and the church.

I wore a dress I already had. I had a simple buffet at home and my next-door neighbor, who was not working at that time, lent me china and silver and helped with the cooking. She was a big help to me; I had no living relatives to invite, so I was very thankful for her comfort and support. She was more excited than I was. I was suffering a case of the last-minute jitters.

Dave and I married during the long Christmas vacation and when we came back to work, Dave went in and told the Personnel Manager. At the same time I went into the lounge during the morning break and told the girls.

It was a complete surprise to everyone and the news spread like wildfire. About half an hour later one of the men in

Dave's unit said, "There's a rumor coming out of the girl's lounge that you and Louise got married. You'd better get out there and stop it." Dave said, "But it's true." And his co-worker choked.

He was one of the men who used to call me "Plain Jane" when the men got together and discussed the women. They had nicknames for most of the girls. Dave had told me about my nickname, but it didn't hurt my feelings. I just laughed. I knew I might look a little dowdy those days, but when younger I'd had a nice figure and average looks. I could look good now, too, if I had time and money to spend on clothes and make-up. I still had a nice figure, but when you buy baggy clothes from K-Mart maybe Plain Jane is the best you can expect. But at that point in time my object in life was maintaining my home and taking care of my sons, not being a sexpot.

The news of our marriage caused a big flap among the supervisors, because company policy had to be checked to see if a married couple could work in the same department. This turned out to be a big question.

To explain: at X Mfg. some large departments were subdivided into sections, and occasionally sections were divided into units. It depended on where the bulk of the work fell. Ours was a large department and had two sections, and one of these sections had two units. We were in a unit. It was determined that it was up to the manager of the section. Our section manager felt it was best to split us up. Accordingly, I switched jobs with a secretary who worked in the other section. This was a lateral transfer, which meant I would not lose my grade or my pay level. It was on the same floor, but on the other side of the building.

Dave was on the management level, but he was not a manager. (Sounds odd, but that's how it was.) His job was titled Parts Pricing Administrator. He had his own office, but it was not one of the enclosed plush corner offices. Only three of the top managers had such offices. His office was small and had partitioned walls that did not reach the ceiling; this meant voices floated and you had to be careful what you said. Nevertheless Dave's office was all his own, with a door he could close. Sometimes he would entice me there on lunch hour so he could close the door and kiss me.

Years later, after I developed my cancer, Dave's office came in handy. Naturally, I could no longer go out to lunch. There was not one restaurant in the entire area that served my kind of food. We packed my lunch — and his. He could have BREAD AND COFFEE, the lucky dog — and at lunchtime we'd go into his office and close the door. Kissing was no longer the reason for closing the door. It was to keep people from barging in to ask work-related questions, but mainly to keep them from asking, WHAT is that STUFF you're eating?

As far as I know, no one ever guessed about my cancer. They may have been suspicious, but I think not. Certain of them were blunt persons who would have said so at once.

It was difficult to explain my diet, on any terms, because drugs and surgery were the usual answers. It was almost a commonplace for employees to take time off for surgical operations. In the girl's lounge there was a pile of women's magazines full of articles that reinforced the common perception that doctors were wonderful heroes who struggled to save you, that operations were easy and wonderful, that Miss Big Star had one and recovered just like nothing, that wonderful new discoveries were coming in by the dozens.

I recall one of the big women's magazines had articles on Marvella Bayh, the Senator's wife, who suffered from breast cancer and had a mastectomy and all the rest. She eventually died, but the way the stories were written made me want to vomit. Here again, the doctor was the big strong silent hero who offered her the best and latest techniques and was so understanding. Mrs. Bayh questioned nothing, she went along, meekly, like a lamb. And everyone in the hospital treated her so nicely, and Mrs. Bayh herself was so BRAVE despite the pain and fear. Pain and fear? Why, the stories made it seem like she was having a picnic!

So, there I was at X Mfg., where many co-workers went off and had operations and came back six or eight weeks later. There I was, claiming to have avoided the worst effects of my colitis by diet.

I felt like an oddball, and this was difficult to contend with. But it was far easier than revealing my cancer and being subjected to their pity. Anything was better than that.

CHAPTER VII

The Diet Itself

One of the thorniest problems I've had while writing this book is deciding whether or not to include the diet. When I first conceived the book, I thought including it was the natural thing to do. I felt many readers would buy with the expectation of obtaining the diet, and I didn't want to disappoint my readers.

As time went by, however, I realized it might be a very unwise thing to do. Let me explain. When Dr. Goldstein worked out my diet he first took my medical history. He wanted to know all about me. He wanted to know what operations I might have had, what previous illnesses I might have had, pills I was in the habit of taking, whether I'd had chemotherapy or radiation, and so on.

My medical history is not the same as that of others. For example, Dr. G devised a diet that greatly helped a man with loss of kidney function, and for him the amount of protein was different from mine. It had to be figured very carefully. If a reader with a kidney problem reads my book, and takes my diet for his own, there might be too much protein in it and he may be harmed rather than helped.

If you have a serious health problem and are interested in helping yourself through diet, I urge you to seek the assistance of a doctor who is nutritionally oriented. I wish you luck; there are not too many, but their number is growing all the time.

I am going to compromise and will give you the menu for one typical meal, to be consumed in the evening. As follows:

MADE IN JUICER—5 ounces carrot juice, 3 ounces celery juice
MADE IN BLENDER**—8 ounces, consisting of:
        1/2 cucumber, peeled
        1/2 green pepper
        4 or 5 dark green leaves of Romaine lettuce
        1 or two stalks of celery **

        Whole salad, in large pieces to be eaten with the fingers, without dressing
        1 piece raw fruit
        3 ounces nuts, raw, unsalted, **OR**
        5 ounces raw milk unsalted cheddar cheese

** This blended salad looks like a green milkshake. Eat slowly, with a spoon. Also, adjust the quantity of vegetables to yield the required amount. Begin with two ounces of distilled water, which you do not count. Put the celery in last, it is the most resistant to blending.

With regard to the nuts, choose from raw, unsalted filberts, walnuts, cashews, peanuts, and blanched almonds. Chew them slowly.

The following must be adhered to.

Eat the foods in the order listed. Juice first, then blended salad, and so on. "Chew them" carefully, sloshing through the teeth, even the juice. Digestion must begin in the mouth. No table or sea salt is to be used. Romaine and green pepper are crucial to this diet. Head lettuce is not to be used, since, being pale green, it is very low in nutrients.

Later when you are allowed steamed food, avoid these vegetables: asparagus, spinach, radishes, onion. Fruits to avoid: figs, dates, raisins. These foods are strong and make the liver work harder.

Drinking water is to be distilled water only. Drink only when thirsty. The "six glasses of water per day" is not the thing here. Too much water overworks your kidneys. You will be getting lots of water in the raw vegetable juices; it will be the purest water you can find anywhere.

Dr. G suggested we get organically grown carrots. He informed us that they could be obtained at Eastern Market 6:00 A.M. on Thursday mornings. They had to be ordered a week ahead, and came by the case. Since we were both working, and the market was at some distance, it was out of the question for us to be there at 6:00 A.M. He then told us, do the best you can. So we bought our supplies at a nearby vegetable store with a name for carrying quality produce.

The carrots are crucial. They are full of beta-carotene, the greatest cancer battler of them all. Do not exceed the amount of carrot juice as given, and always dilute with another juice, as too much Vitamin A is hard on the liver. Celery juice is good for this purpose, since it is very good for the nerves.

An important statement: the blended salad, as given, lessens the body's need for a more complex protein.

However, I found this to be one of the most difficult new foods to become accustomed to. In the beginning, it tastes bitter. As time goes by, you get used to it. And sometimes when the vegetables have a mild flavor, the blended salad tastes rather nice.

As for fruit, try to concentrate on fruits **WHEN THEY ARE IN SEASON**. They are the cheapest when in season, but more important, they are the most nutritious when eaten at their peak of natural ripeness.

As time went on, Dr. G gradually added items to my diet. Some of them were quite impossible for me to tolerate, such as sprouts and sunflower seeds. These put too much rough-age in my system. He suggested them because of various food values he knew them to contain, and it is a pity I couldn't include them from time to time, at least to provide variety. This lack of variety was a problem I had to contend with for many years. There were times I felt as I did in that infamous Supermarket Incident, when I felt like banging my head on the wall.

Upon one occasion when I complained to him that my colitis would not permit me to eat raw fruits, he told me to eat only the pulpy fruits like banana, papaya, mango, and peaches. Not to eat plums, grapes, cherries, or anything with skins that could not be removed. He also mentioned to avoid all citrus fruits and acid fruits, including pineapple.

On another occasion, he said it was all right to try water-melon, so I did. At that time, though it did not cause actual pain, it did give me tremendous amounts of gas, causing much distention of the abdomen. My bloated belly made me look five pounds heavier than I was. (Dave teased me, say-ing, are you sure you're not pregnant?) Now that I am in a calmer frame of mind and I take care to eat it slowly at the beginning of a meal, I can enjoy watermelon.

I remember asking Dr. G if I could maybe, once in a great while, have a cup of hot chocolate to perk up my spirits. The dismal answer was, "NO!" Dr. G went on to explain why. Lend an ear to this.

Chocolate contains theobromine, a diuretic which takes potassium from the system. It contains caffeine, a stimulant which makes for nervousness. It is partly alkaloid, leading to an imbalance of minerals in the system.

I defy anyone to enjoy his chocolate after learning that!

I was amazed one day when he said I could have honey ice cream now and then. I rushed out and bought some and found, to my distress (but probably to my benefit) that it was so sweet I couldn't stand it.

Here is a listing of food items which are generally good for cancer patients, because of high amounts of B-17: lentils, millet, mung beans, corn, buckwheat, groats, chick peas, brown rice.

Most of these things gave me too much gas. Corn, with its little cellulose jacket on every kernel, almost killed me. Lentils and millet pose a difficult problem, in another way. They are very bland, so much so it is almost impossible to make them tasty, especially when you can't use salt. I devised a few of my own recipes, which I will give you in a later chapter.

At one time Dr. G said I could add oatmeal to my diet. It should be the steel-cut variety, and cooked without salt. Back in 1980, because of relative scarcity of health food stores, it was difficult to find. And without salt or milk, not very exciting. I added cinnamon and nutmeg to the cooking water and a spoonful of honey. This somewhat took the curse off the blandness and provided much-welcomed variety. Also, this dish was very soothing to my tummy, which was in a constant uproar during those early years.

As time went by Dr. G gradually added new items to my diet. These were asparagus, broccoli, spinach, and mushrooms. The first three were to be lightly steamed—unsalted, unbuttered, and unsauced. Hollandaise sauce was out of my life! Mushrooms were to be sliced raw and added to my whole salad. But here again, with these items, too much roughage. These foods were also a lot of bother; cleaning all these fresh vegetables takes time. Oh, for the good old days, when all I did was put a chop or steak on the broiler, toss potatoes in the pressure cooker, open a can of peas, chop a little head lettuce, and with expenditure of very little time, had a meal ready.

I am often asked three things about my diet.

What is wrong with meat?
Why is milk to be avoided?
What is wrong with cooked food?

For the answer to the question about meat, I refer you to pages 212 and 213 of Dr. Goldstein's book. To quote some of what he says, here are the following passages:
"The meat and starches tend to stagnate in the intestinal tract, since they do not stimulate intestinal motility to evacuate them. As a result, there are poisonous waste products from the putrefaction of these "hung-up" foods, which come in contact with the intestinal lining regularly and for prolonged periods."

And: "The end products of meat digestion and putrefaction in the intestinal tract are such poisons as skatol, indol, phenol, acetic acid, and uric acid, all of which tend to poison the body. The uric acid is responsible for gout and gouty arthritis as well as kidney stones."

As for milk (cow's milk, that is) his chief objection to it is that it is for the digestive system of the calf, not the human baby. It is an acid-forming food, has more fat, and so is harder for us to digest. Human enzymes will not break down the protein in cow's milk. Mother's milk is better because it is tailor-made for the human baby, whereas cow's milk is made for the calf. Furthermore, when cow's milk is pasteurized (as it must be for fear of tuberculous cows) it is ruined, because enzymes are destroyed. It also forms mucus and leads to stuffy sinuses and congested lungs.

Goat's milk would be better for the infant. I tried goat's milk and I know why cow's milk is preferred. Goat's milk is a dirty gray color, unappetizing to look at, and has an awful taste. That's when I realized that cow's milk is so widely popular because it is, basically, sweet tasting.

I asked Dr. G if cow's milk might not help ease my colitis. He said No, in fact, it could cause colitis. This is due to the fact that in the adult human the enzyme, renin, which curdles the milk to enable its digestion, is present in very limited amounts. He stressed the point that animals never return to milk once they mature. Man is the only mammal who does. In years back, this was probably because cow's milk was a cheap, easily available food. Nowadays, it is probably because the Milk Producers' Association runs colorful spots on television, showing attractive vigorous people enjoying glasses of sparkling white milk.

I realize it is difficult to accept this information about milk. It seems to be part of the very fabric of our lives. I fed it to my sons when they were infants so they'd have strong bones and teeth. My grandmother would not give me milk when I was a child, because she was afraid of tuberculosis in cows. Cows are very susceptible to this disease. At any rate, I had very poor teeth and blamed it on lack of milk while I was growing up.

Dr. G also mentioned that milk and wheat are very common allergens, but many people never realize it. This is because the symptoms are only mildly distressing and often laid to the door of something else.

The third question is: What is wrong with cooked food? I will make short hash of this. Cooked food is dead food. Minerals, vitamins and enzymes are destroyed. I realize that certain vegetables, grains, etc., must be cooked to be edible, but they should form only fifty per cent or so of our diet.

Wheat is extremely difficult to eliminate from the ordinary diet. Bread, toast, crackers, bagels, Danish rolls, cakes, cookies, and pies all contain wheat flour. Rye bread is not a good substitute, as it contains at least 50 per cent wheat flour in order to keep it from being too heavy and "damp" inside.

Additives, additives. Commonly called, junk foods. For a listing of additives that will dazzle your mind and keep your awake at nights, I refer you to Chapter IX of Dr. Goldstein's book. I'm going to quote from page 186:

"Sodium Benzoate — a deadly poison used as a preservative in soda pop, jams, jellies, pickles, and countless other so-called foods. Speaking of soda, caffeine is used in all cola drinks. The concerned parent who forbids the child the ingestion of coffee or tea unknowingly allows the child to consume enormous amounts of caffeine when the unlimited use of cola drinks is permitted. Sodium Benzoate kills or inhibits all living organisms present within the jar or other container. We are living organisms, too, but the harmful effects, because of small doses in food products, don't make themselves evident until years later."

He makes the point that many artificial colors and flavors are coal-tar derivatives, and these are cancer-causing.

When you have finished reading this chapter, you may react as I did. I wondered how our government, in the form of the Food and Drug Administration, could have let such a situation arise, that most of the things on grocery shelves are harmful to us. What are we paying them for? How do they operate?

It is my hope that someone among my readers who is younger and stronger than I might begin to agitate for some housecleaning at the FDA.

CHAPTER VIII

Recipes and Cooking Tips

BROWN RICE   Benefits are: it has good protein value, and the eight essential amino acids are well proportioned. It is anti-cancer and speaking for myself, I notice it is good for the nerves.

There are different varieties, and cooking instructions may vary. In general, however, this is what works.

        1 cup brown rice
        2 cups distilled water
        1 tablespoon cold-pressed soy oil
        1/2 teaspoon sea salt, if desired

        Rice: if necessary, pick out black or deformed
                grains
        Water: use distilled
        Oil: any unsaturated, cold-pressed oil will do;
                keeps grains from sticking together
        Salt: use sea salt. If salt is forbidden to you,
                replace with 1 tablespoon parsley, dry or
                fresh, and a mashed garlic clove

Place ingredients in DEEP PAN with TIGHT FITTING LID. Repeat, TIGHT LID. Stir. Cover tightly. Bring rapidly to boil; remove from heat, allow burner to cool to medium, replace, simmer slowly forty minutes. Check for water level.

Add an ounce or so, if needed to prevent scorching. Simmer another five minutes or so. Test. Should be a bit crunchy. Serve at once.

DRIED BEANS AND LENTILS These need to be soaked over night, and next day will require two hours cooking time. Do not attempt to short cut by using pressure cooker; they will froth up, make a dreadful mess on your stove, and might even blow up.

If you forgot to soak them, cover with water, cover tightly, bring quickly to boil, remove from heat, let stand two hours. Cook in same water for additional two hours.

LENTIL SOUP This will be more flavorful if you have a chicken carcass to use for a base. Chicken should be hormone free, of course. I use the bones for lentil soup after I have roasted the bird and eaten the meat at an earlier meal. I do this to get my money's worth; hormone-free birds are so expensive. If you have no bones, there will be no chicken flavor, so use chicken bouillon from the health food store; be careful it has no salt. Do not use the bouillon, loose or in cubes, from the supermarket. This will be too salty; also it will be derived from poultry that has been raised with hormones.

LENTIL SOUP

> 1 1/2 cups lentils, washed (12 ounces)
> 1 1/2 quarts water
> 1/2 teaspoon salt
> 1/4 teaspoon thyme
> 1 teaspoon ground celery seed
> Bones from one medium-size chicken, and
>   giblets (which have been boiled for three
>   minutes and rinsed well)

Wash lentils, pick over, drain. Combine with all ingredients above, except the bones and giblets. Place in cooking kettle, cover, soak overnight on top of stove.

Next day, ADD one medium onion, chopped. Add bones and giblets, cover tightly, and simmer SLOWLY for two hours, in same water. Stir occasionally. Then add:

> 1 small can stewed tomatoes (14.5 ounces), or
> 2 fresh peeled tomatoes
> 2–3 carrots, diced about 1/4 inch
> 1 medium potato, diced

and simmer for twenty minutes.

The lentils will more than double in size. You may omit the carrots and potato, but add the tomatoes; they give a nice brown color.

PASTA

If there is a dead food that is deader than pasta, I can't imagine what it is. Consider these facts: first, the flour is milled and processed, and to make it fine and white, all the health-giving bran is removed. Second, it is mixed with egg and salt and water and rolled out into pasta, then dried and cut. Thirdly, it is then boiled. Anything that has been handled three successive times simply cannot retain very much value, in terms of a food that is nutritious for the body.

However, having said that, for those among you who love Italian food and need a little time to wean yourself away, here's a little help.

VEGETARIAN PASTA

Go to the health food store and buy some of the new varieties that are available now. Plan ahead to make the sauce early in the day, or the day before.

MEATLESS SPAGHETTI SAUCE

6 ounces fresh mushrooms (wipe them off
    with a damp cloth and slice)
1/2 fresh green pepper, diced
1 medium yellow onion, chopped
4 garlic cloves, minced
1 1/2 large jars tomato sauce, meatless, of
    course, about 32 ounces
1/4 cup water
1/2 teaspoon dry basil, crushed
1/8 teaspoon black pepper

Saute the first four items in a little cold-pressed oil in a heavy pan till onions are yellow. The mushrooms will produce a lot of water. Add remaining ingredients, cover tightly, simmer slowly one hour, stirring occasionally. Let stand several hours before using. If you wish to keep it overnight, to give the flavors more time to blend, transfer to a stainless steel pan and place in refrigerator. The mushrooms are crunchy like meat and if you don't tell people there's no meat in the dish, they won't even miss it.

Incidentally, DON'T USE ALUMINUM PANS OR PRESSURE COOKERS. GET RID OF ANY YOU MAY HAVE.

People used to laugh at the old wives' tale that aluminum pans might cause cancer, but here is some shocking news. Mr. Earl Mindell, who wrote the VITAMIN BIBLE and other books, recently said that aluminum has been found in the brain cells of victims of Alzheimer's Disease. How's that for some awful news? The local doctor who was his radio host immediately challenged Mr. Mindell and said, "Has it been PROVEN there is a definite link?" And Mr. Mindell replied, "No, but I'm not waiting ten years for a definitive study to come out, I'm staying away from the stuff." Substances to avoid, Mr. Mindell said, are roll-on deodorants, aluminum foil, antacids, processed cheese. Can you imagine a manufacturer using aluminum to process cheese? I call that the height of irresponsibility. That manufacturer must think of profit only. Where, oh where, is the food company that has a social conscience?

Mr. Mindell added that aluminum content is not, **repeat not**, always marked on the labels.

SOYBEANS

Soybeans are often hailed as a cheap source of protein. True, but they are also exceptionally bland. I spent the better part of a year experimenting with them, trying to give them flavor. They have to be soaked overnight first, and I tried soaking them in every combination of garlic, spices, you name it, I tried it. The only thing that will give them flavor is mixing them with meat, and when you can't eat meat, forget the soybeans.

ROAST CHICKEN

You must find birds that are raised without hormones. If you live near any Amish farmers, in their market town you may find hormone-free chickens. Otherwise, go to a health food store.

To prepare, remove giblets, rinse inside and out. Remove any feathers and chunks of fat. Pat dry with paper towels. Sprinkle inside with sea salt and poultry seasoning, also the chest cavity.

Take a medium onion, peel it, cut in half (or into quarters if the bird is small). Take a large stalk of celery, cut into pieces to fit. Place celery and onion inside. Peel a garlic clove, cut it in half, slip under the breast skin.

Cut a piece of clean white cloth, such as a linen dishtowel, to fit over breast and legs. Put bird on rack in roasting pan, place in oven preheated to 325 degrees F. Melt about 1/4 cup unsalted butter in small pan, dip cloth into it, then place on bird. Every 20 minutes dip small brush into melted butter and apply to cloth. If you don't have a suitable pastry brush, you may use a clean 1 inch paint brush, unused for paint, of course; or you may use the back of a big spoon to keep the butter from running right off.

For the last one-third of the cooking time, use a baster (bulb syringe type) to suck up juices from bottom of roasting pan, and baste bird every 20 minutes. This produces a juicy bird with a pleasant roasted flavor.

The average 3 to 3 1/2 pound chicken will cook in 1 1/2 to 2 hours; a bird that is 4 to 5 pounds will cook in 2 1/2 to 3 hours. Over 5 pounds, 3 to 4 hours.

In view of what we just learned from Mr. Mindell, I will not include instructions about cooking the bird in aluminum foil.

If you are worried about cholesterol, which I am not (being on this diet keeps my level low) you may use soy oil to brush the bird and baste it with a cloth dipped in white wine. Be sure the wine is not too strong. For continuing basting, boil up a cup of water with some garlic, parsley, and black peppercorns. Boil it down to one-half. Start this mixture before you begin preparing the fowl.

For gravy, remove bird to warm platter and cover with clean brown paper and then a terry cloth towel. Carefully pour drippings from roasting pan into small pan and reheat, and use them in place of gravy.

LOW CALORIE WAY TO BROIL FISH

Cod, sole, or haddock from North Atlantic waters is recommended as being cleanest. Defrost immediately before use. Sole may require only twenty minutes, depending on how it is packaged. Rinse in cold water. Rub a wedge of lemon or lime over all sides. Dry on paper towels. Stronger fish such as red snapper should be soaked in a shallow bowl of milk for half an hour to remove the strong taste. When fish is defrosted, if it has an offensive "fishy" smell, it is not safe to be eaten and should be discarded. That's why it's a good practice to use frozen fish soon after purchase; it's easier to take it back to the store and demand a refund.

Grease heavily a glass casserole dish, 8 inch by 8 inch by 2 inch, with oil. Place fillets in dish. Do NOT overlap. If your family is bigger and you need two packages, use a 9 x 13 x 2 inch dish.

For one package, heat in small pan:

> 1/4 cup cold-pressed oil
> Add juice of 1/4 lemon, stir

Pour over fish. In electric oven, broil-bake at 450 degrees F. with door closed. Cook 10 to 15 minutes. Baste once half-way through the cooking time. When done, apply softened butter and sprinkle with paprika.

As soon as you put it in the oven, begin warming up the serving platter.

Fish will be cooked through when it turns white and flakes easily with a fork. Be sure it is done. While getting it ready, if you're preparing sole and some of it is thin, leave thinner pieces out for the first five minutes. Otherwise they will burn and get dry while you cook the thicker pieces. When you take it out, look it over thoroughly. If any portion looks transparent, it is not cooked, return to oven for a few minutes.

On the other hand, do not overcook. It will get dry. Serve at once. This means you must have other dishes under way, and table set. (In fact, a good general practice before meals is to set the table completely first, select serving dishes, figure out the various cooking times, and begin cooking with the items that take longest.)

FISH SAUCE

This is similar to tartar sauce, but is home made.

> 2/3 cup mayonnaise, from a health food store
> 2 tablespoons milk, more or less, to make the
>   sauce a little thin
> 1 tablespoon capers, drained and minced
> 1 tablespoon onion, minced finely
> 1 tablespoon fresh parsley, minced with
>   scissors, or 1/2 tablespoon dried parsley
>   flakes

Mix ahead in small bowl, one nice enough to use for serving, cover tightly, and let stand in refrigerator at least six hours. Advise your family to place it next to the fish, rather than on top, to avoid chilling the fish before it can be eaten.

Capers may be found in tiny jars in the specialty section of the supermarket.

For a decalorized version, for the mayonnaise substitute:

> 1/3 cup plain yogurt
> 1/3 cup mayonnaise
> (milk not necessary)

VEGETABLE BROTH

Dr. Goldstein gave me this recipe as one of the first cooked dishes I was allowed. It is very beneficial for a body weakened by cancer or other illness, since it could also be called "Potassium Broth." Needless to say, all vegetables must be fresh.

> 2 fresh peeled tomatoes, cut in 1/8
> 1 small zucchini or more, 1/2 inch slices
> 1 large carrot, 1/4 inch slices
> 1 medium potato, cut in 1/6

2 parsnips, in 3/8 inch dices
2 medium onion, chopped coarsely
3 stalks celery, 1 inch pieces
1/2 green pepper, 1 inch pieces
Parsley, fresh, snipped, about 1 tablespoon
1 cup green beans, in 1 inch pieces, added last
6-8 fresh basil leaves, if available

When vegetables are cut, place in a large bowl, except for the green beans. To get the correct measurement of water, cover the vegetables with distilled water, then add one more cup. Pour water off, into deep pan with tight-fitting lid, bring to boil. Add vegetables. Cook 5 minutes. Add green beans, cook five more minutes or so.

Remove from heat, keep covered, let stand ten minutes. Pour off the broth, drink it, and discard the vegetables. You will be drinking a big "mineral tablet" with all the minerals in good balance, in a form your body will be able to utilize at once.

If you have a problem with discarding the vegetables, after all the work of preparing them, you might make a soup. What I do now that I feel my health is good, is the following. I get a can of sodium-free tomato sauce, heat it up, sprinkle in some grated parmesan cheese, let the cheese melt in, and add some of the vegetables.

If you try this recipe, be sure to include the parsnips. They add a sweet flavor. As for the parsley, it does a great deal to compensate for the lack of salt.

NOTE: In general, two minced garlic cloves and 1 table-spoon of parsley are a good salt substitute in certain dishes.

ZUCCHINI

I understand in Italy they pick zucchini and other summer squash when the size of small pickles, then promptly cook in a frying pan with a little butter. In the United States markets sell them at five or six inches in size. Home gardeners may let them grow larger, but six to eight inches is the largest that is recommended, for they will become rather woody and tasteless.

> 2 zucchini, six inches long
> 4–6 large mushrooms (optional)
> 1/2 medium onion, chopped
> 1/2 green pepper, chopped
> 1 tablespoon soy oil, or other mild
>   cold-pressed oil

Wipe mushrooms with a damp cloth, slice, chop into half-inch pieces. Cut zucchini into 1/4 inch slices, then chop into 1/2 inch pieces.

Warm up a heavy frying pan, add the oil. Saute mushrooms, onion and green pepper at medium heat for 5 minutes, keeping covered, turning occasionally. Add zucchini, continue cooking for 5 to 8 minutes, just until zucchini tests tender when pierced with a fork.

I do not advise boiling zucchini in water. It gets overdone very fast. Steaming is better, if you have a steamer that works correctly. The above recipe gives it flavor and crunch. Zucchini is very low in calories, yet high in potassium and vitamin A.

* * * *

I hope you find my recipes interesting and helpful. They are a start, at least, to a more healthful way of cooking.

CHAPTER IX

The Keystone to Health — Your Liver

Many times during my first few years on this diet, I found myself longing for more variety. Knowing some of the limitations, I would put my mind to work trying to think of something that might be acceptable. I would then call up Dr. Goldstein and put the proposition to him. Almost every time he would say, "No, it's too hard on your liver."

After several of these incidents, I began to wonder what it was about the liver that made it so special. I had seen many articles about cholesterol, but never a word did I see about the liver. It was doing something important, but what?

I went to my local library and they didn't think much of the liver either—they didn't have one listing in their card catalog. I went to a slightly larger library, there again, nothing.

I began calling libraries in other suburbs, and there again, nothing. At last a librarian suggested I look into medical encyclopedias in the reference section. In them I did find a little information, but not enough.

Determined to find more, I borrowed some medical textbooks from my chiropractor, Dr. Dan Laframboise. He gave me three, and they were such big books I could barely stagger out of the office with them. Unfortunately, although the writing style was clear, there were lots of big words that made the language as heavy as the books. I had to read these books many times before I could understand them.

I will try to put together some of what I've learned to help you understand the liver.

The Liver has more than
500
separate functions

The largest of our organs, the liver is about twelve inches long and weighs about three pounds. It lies in the uppermost part of the right side of the abdomen. The lower edge can be felt in front of your body, just under the ribs on your right side.

The liver is, in fact, about the size of a football and it is a reddish-brown color, like many footballs are.

If you were to remove something from your body the size of a football, you'd certainly notice the hole that was left.

As you will see on the page which lists functions of the liver, metabolism is mentioned often.

Metabolism is the sum total of the many chemical processes in the body which use food and transform it so that the body can use it in the cells.

Dr. Fishbein's Medical Encyclopedia says, on page 1921, that:

"Because body tissue is constantly being destroyed, synthesis of new tissue is a vital function of metabolism."

What it all boils down to is this: since the liver is vitally involved in metabolism, it is especially important to good nutrition, AND keeping the immune system fit.

Therefore, if the body has been weakened by a serious illness or bad habits of a lifetime, and you want to restore health, then the easier you can make things for your liver, the better off you are.

The liver is further remarkable in that it can "rebuild" itself if it has been damaged. This means that if the causes of the damage are removed, the liver can rebuild itself—providing, of course, the damage has not gone too far.

You can make it easier for your liver to heal or to stay healthy by getting lots of REST and by NOT taking the following:

> alcohol
> nicotine
> caffeine
> meat
> white sugar
> white flour
> fatty foods
> chocolate

Caffeine: Please remember most cola drinks contain caffeine, as do many teas.

Fatty foods: Please be aware that fast foods should be kept to a minimum. For example, the chicken sandwiches which have recently become popular in fast food restaurants in the United States in the mid-1980's are breaded and then fried in beef fat—which makes them very tasty, but does increase cholesterol.

White sugar: This includes Danish pastry and doughnuts as well as cookies, candy bars, and all the usual sweets. People often turn to honey and molasses and brown sugar, but these are also sugars that give lots of work to the liver.

Other foods that are hard on the liver are strong vegetables such as broccoli, asparagus, and spinach; and dried fruits, because of the concentrated sugars in them.

As for getting lots of rest, this is what I sometimes, in a mood of cynicism, call "garbage advice." Meaning, "Easier said than Done." Our lives today are so stressful, so fragmented, and so pressed for time, that it is difficult to find time to rest. Even if you do manage to lie down or sit in your favorite easy chair, you still may not be able to relax. I will give some suggestions on stress and time management in a later chapter.

Other things you can do to keep your liver healthy are to be moderate in eating and drinking, and avoid chemicals, additives, and processed foods as much as possible. Try to eat foods that are close to the natural state. An ancient Greek school of philosophy recommended moderation in all things, and it's still a good idea.

But before we leave our discussion of that quiet, dependable workhorse, the human liver, let me sum up:

Be kind to your liver,

It is vital to the health of your body.

BASIC LIVER FUNCTIONS—AT A GLANCE

Makes glucose (fuel)
from food, stores it

Releases fuel to muscles
for energy

Makes bile for
digestion of fats

Sends bile back and forth
to gall bladder, as needed

Turns certain amino acids
into protein for the blood

Maintains balance
of the hormones

Stores Iron, Copper,
and certain vitamins

Collects and excretes
various wastes

Neutralizes and excretes poisons,
thus cleansing the blood

Regulates clotting
of the blood

CHAPTER **X**

Home and Herbal Remedies

As I mentioned earlier, at various times I have been laid low by serious ailments. I knew I could not take antibiotics or antihistamines or other drugs to help.

How did I know?

Dr. Goldstein told me that keeping chemicals out of my body was one of the cornerstones of his plan.

There is yet another way I knew. Back in the summer of 1978, about six months after I learned of my cancer, I was still working and having a bad time on the job. I had gotten a new supervisor and as I have mentioned, he was mean and manipulative. Dr. G would not prescribe a tranquilizer so I, feeling ready to fall apart from unhappiness and frustration, went to another doctor and got a prescription for Valium.

I took the Valium for several days, and my nerves felt immensely better. I was able to go to work and control my desire to confront my boss and tell him he was a terrible person.

Taking this drug, however, proved to be a mistake. A new lump appeared in my breast almost immediately. For me, this was undeniable proof that chemicals are bad for the body.

I quit taking the Valium, continued my raw diet, got more rest, and within a week the lump disappeared.

This, to me, was a miracle — a miracle of my own body.

From that point on, I never even considered taking any

drugs. Whenever I became ill, I turned to home and herbal remedies. If I couldn't find something suitable, I just suffered it out and went to bed earlier.

One of my sources for herbal remedies was the old book, BACK TO EDEN, written years ago by Jethro Kloss, who helped many people with his herb doctoring. The book is badly written and badly organized, but because basically the information is good, it is still in print.

In Chapter Five he mentions fasting, which means drinking only water and eating no food. BEWARE OF WATER FASTING IF YOU HAVE CANCER. Dr. Goldstein told me that although it can help people with certain ailments such as colitis and arthritis, water fasting can kill a cancer patient very quickly.

Fasting by way of juices, however, is an entirely different thing. It can be very beneficial to a cancer patient. The juices should be freshly made from raw vegetables in the proper combinations.

For two winters in a row, both times in the month of January, I was seriously ill with lung flu. Mr. Kloss' book suggested drinking hot water with lemon juice in it while taking a hot bath and then going straight to bed with the covers piled on. The dose I used was one cup of hot (distilled) water with one teaspoon of fresh lemon juice.

(I do not use the bottled, concentrated, or frozen juice. I do not feel that anything that is processed has as much life as it had before.)

I found this practice very helpful. I do not say that it hastened my cure, as I have no way of knowing this, but it did ease my symptoms and made me feel I was doing something to help myself.

About lemon juice (meaning FRESH lemon juice, of course) Mr. Kloss explains its curative properties as follows:

"It is an antiseptic, or is an agent that will prevent sepsis or putrefaction. It is also anti-scorbutic, the term meaning a remedy which will prevent disease and assist in cleansing the system of impurities. The lemon is a wonderful stimulant to the liver and is a dissolvent of uric acid and other poisons, liquifies the bile, and is very good in cases of malaria."

Notice the reference to lemon as being a wonderful stimulant to the liver.

Mr. Kloss also mentions that lemon juice should NEVER be taken with sugar, and that is most helpful when taken an hour before meals, on an empty stomach.

This last instruction is not easy to follow. It takes a lot of planning. If you are at work, it cannot be done, unless you plan enough ahead to take the mixture with you in a thermos bottle. It is a little easier to do at home, of course, but it still requires planning and determination.

Upon another occasion, I suffered bladder problems. I couldn't tell whether or not I had to urinate and when I tried, it was very difficult to start. Once started, it was difficult to empty the bladder completely.

Several times a day, half an hour before meals, I drank hot water and lemon juice. I took care to drink it as hot as I could stand it. I also voided promptly whenever the urge came. Within a week or so, my bladder was back to normal.

Mr. Kloss was a great believer in the curative power of water. Baths and foot soaks are frequently mentioned. We all know the skin excretes by means of sweating, but we have lost sight of a few other facts. One, that it excretes poisons through the pores in general, and two, that it absorbs. For example, if you were to throw a handful of herbs into your bath, your skin would absorb the beneficial properties of that particular herb.

Some people think the skin doesn't absorb. If it doesn't, why do dermatologists use a variety of potions and ointments?

Mr. Kloss stresses that water should be the purest that can be obtained. Unfortunately, with our city water systems as they are, it is impossible to get pure water for taking baths, but it helps to add one cup of apple cider vinegar.

The vinegar softens the water, invigorates the body, and soothes the skin. The skin, being a protein, should be slightly acid. When I want to get started fast in the mornings, I throw in a cup of vinegar, have the water warm but not hot, and rub very vigorously while in the tub.

However, for drinking, let me tell you about an experiment conducted by the Natural Hygiene Society, Detroit chapter, which occurred about fifteen years ago. A distillation apparatus was brought to the meeting place, and at the beginning of the meeting five gallons of Detroit city water were poured in.

By the end of the meeting, the water had gone through the distiller. The residue looked like sewer sludge; it simply turned everyone's stomach. The people in attendance decided to buy distilled water for drinking and cooking purposes.

In January of 1981 I went to a meeting of a mystery writer's group at the home of one of the members. The scheduled speaker was a detective from the Homicide Squad of the Detroit Police Department. He talked for two hours and his stories were so fascinating that we all sat riveted in attention.

We were gathered in a rather small living room with no ventilation. One man was smoking a cigarillo and another a pipe. The time passed so quickly we never realized how thickly the smoke was piling up.

When I reached home, I realized my head was full of smoke. The next morning my sinuses were badly clogged and I had a dreadful headache which lasted several days. I had great difficulty breathing and lost my appetite.

Unwilling to use antihistamines because of their chemical content, I consulted BACK TO EDEN once again and decided to use the herb, comfrey, to ease my symptoms. The only form available at the time was the root, ground up and placed in capsules, from the health food store.

I received some relief from them. However, the following summer I visited a new friend and mentioned my problem to her. She told me she had a comfrey plant growing in her rock garden, and she gave me some fresh leaves.

I took them home and made tea. Upon drinking the tea, freshly made and steaming hot, I experienced greater and faster relief. Through this experience, I realized first hand that in this case, at any rate, tea made from fresh leaves was far more effective than dried root put into capsules.

Later on my friend gave me a stem off her plant. I took it home and rooted it and since then have grown it in my garden. I still suffer from an allergy to smoke. When I am exposed to it socially, I come home and brew the tea and find relief right away. This has two benefits: it is a cheap way to go, and I don't have to put chemicals into my system.

As I mentioned in Chapter Four, I have occasionally taken a coffee enema to help speed up getting poisons out of my system. Dr. Goldstein is not in favor of them, because he feels they deplete the system of minerals. However, after a trip abroad, for instance, when I've been forced to eat questionable foods, I feel they are helpful.

Here's how it is done. Preheat the enema bag by filling it with hot water. In the bathroom spread a heavy piece of plastic on the floor, cover it with a beach towel. Fold up a bath towel to put under your head.

In the kitchen, bring to a boil two cups of distilled water. Add four teaspoons of instant coffee. Stir, and add two cups of distilled water (room temperature). This will make the water tepid, just right for use. Empty the enema bag, fill with the coffee mixture, and grease the tip with vaseline.

Wearing only an old pajama top (and socks if your feet get cold easily) lie down on your right side, draw up your knees, relax your tummy, and begin letting the coffee mixture in. At first you won't be able to retain the fluid for very long, but near the end of the session, try to retain about a cup of the coffee mixture for five minutes.

Dr. Harold Manner, of the Metabolic Research Foundation, formerly of Glenview, Illinois, recommends holding one cup for fifteen minutes, but I find that impossible. Do the best you can. Try to schedule this early in the day. If you do it in the evening, the effects of the caffeine may have you merrily scrubbing the floor at ten o'clock in the evening.

My husband, David, who stood by me staunchly throughout my cancer experience, is a very loving person. I found that repeated use of contraceptive foam was giving me a continuing case of vaginitis. Since I couldn't go to a gynecologist and get an Rx for medicine, I tried using that old standby, the vinegar douche. This was of very little help.

I tried one-half cup of plain yogurt mixed with one pint of water, using it twice a day as a douche. In eight or ten days the condition was cleared up. I also gave up wearing shorts and slacks, and cut small holes in my pantyhose and panties so there wouldn't be that build-up of heat which contributes to vaginitis. These two methods were very helpful. I am no longer bothered by this problem.

However, in a cold climate, it's a nuisance not to be able to wear slacks to keep your legs warm. In the winter I wear long woolen skirts and leg warmers to compensate, and in the summer I wear cotton skirts, rather than shorts. Not an ideal state of affairs, but at least it's better than being troubled by a constant itch.

I notice doctors are now advising young men who may be having fertility problems not to wear tight jockey shorts or jeans. A build-up of heat is the problem here also.

In my family there is a tendency to develop keloid scars when there is a bad cut. Keloid means when the scar tissue raises a lump above the skin. About two years after I developed the cancer, I found a mole on my shoulder just under my bra strap. It grew as big as a dime and was irritated by the strap. I went to my general practitioner and he removed it. In time, it healed, but with a big keloid lump.

He sent me to a dermatologist. I explained my anti-cancer program to him, stating very clearly I didn't want anything done without talking it over. He agreed, then looked at the keloid lump and — surprise? — without another word shot it full of cortisone. When I protested, he said blithely it wouldn't interfere with my anti-cancer program. He gave me another shot the following week and told me to come in for one more. The lump did reduce in size somewhat, but I also got another lump — in my breast.

Needless to say, I did not return for the third shot, and now I had TWO lumps. The lump in my breast gradually went away and my skepticism about medication increased.

However, the lump on my shoulder was disfiguring and I still wanted to get rid of it. I read somewhere (can't remember where) that sometimes castor oil will reduce this type of scar. Twice a day I applied a hot wet wash cloth to the scar for a few minutes, then rubbed in a little castor oil. It took over two months, as best I can recall, but eventually the scar flattened out.

One more victory without medication.

I still suffer from colitis periodically. By this I mean excessive gassiness in the abdomen, sometimes with pain, sometimes not, but very seldom with diarrhea. Being very suspicious of all medications, including over the counter gas relievers because they generally contain aluminum, I can't obtain quick comfort by taking one of these popular preparations.

Here are some of my home remedies. Please remember I always use distilled water for drinking and making teas. I find the following ways helpful to relieve the discomfort from gas:

1) A cup of hot water, plain
2) A cup of hot water, boiled for a few
   minutes in a small pan with a teaspoon of
   raw honey
3) The above, with one teaspoon of cider
   vinegar added
4) Caraway Seed infusion

The first three are very good for getting up burps. The Caraway Seed tea is helpful for soothing the entire digestive system and eliminating gas from the intestines. Here is my recipe for it:

CARAWAY SEED TEA

2 heaping tablespoons Caraway Seeds
2 cups distilled water
2 tablespoons honey

Use stainless steel or glass pan only, with a tight-fitting lid. Bring the water to a boil. Add the honey, using one spoon. Let honey dissolve, then using another spoon, add the caraway seeds. (If you add honey first and use only one spoon, you will have a sticky mess to deal with.) Cover tightly, gently boil for five minutes. Remove from heat, let stand covered for 15 minutes. Strain, sip one-half of the drink, move around, get on your bed and do the knee-chest exercise (the one women do after giving birth) about five times. Drink rest of tea. I always feel immensely better after doing this. This mixture is very soothing to the digestive system.

I used to have a copy of the book, FOLK MEDICINE, by the New England country doctor, D. C. Jarvis. I no longer have my copy, and I think he may have been a veterinarian. At any rate, he tells about the usefulness of various home remedies, and he gives a great deal of space to the benefits of cider vinegar.

When I entered my menopause, I scarcely knew it. Apparently being on this carefully designed diet given me by Dr. Goldstein straightened out my system so that my hormones responded with little fuss. I had very few hot flashes and only a few irregular periods. I did have some general discomfort and mentioned this to my chiropractor, Dr. Dan LaFramboise.

Dr. Dan suggested drinking a glass of warm water with a teaspoon of cider vinegar in it, three times a day, I added a spoonful of honey, and found almost instant relief when I began sipping it.

I mentioned this to Dr. Goldstein and he said it was okay to drink vinegar upon occasion, but he couldn't recommend it as a regular part of my diet because vinegar is fermented, and as such puts a little extra strain on the liver. As we know from my earlier chapter, Dr. G is very much concerned with the welfare of the liver.

Other fermented items to beware of are pickles, wine, beer, liquor, liqueurs. I am permitted an occasional glass of white wine.

To say a little more about vinegar, I began collecting notes on its many household uses. (I don't use white vinegar because I discovered it receives extra processing which I don't approve of.) Here are some of its uses:

Deodorize the cat box by rinsing with vinegar. Remove salt stains on shoes and boots, using equal parts vinegar and water. Eliminate fresh paint and wall paper paste fumes by placing small bowls of vinegar in the room. Eliminate onion odors on your hands. Remove lime deposits around water faucets and shower heads. Soak a paper towel and lay it over the faucets. For showerheads, I fill a plastic bag with vinegar and tie it tightly over the head and leave it on for at least twelve hours.

Remove grease and odors from kitchen stove, etc., by adding a few tablespoons to the cleaning water. It is far less smelly than ammonia. I can't use ammonia or chlorine bleach any more because of my sinuses being so damaged from that smoke allergy I told you about earlier in this chapter. Vinegar is a good substitute for ammonia and bleach, and so is baking soda.

This is how I clean the drain in my kitchen sink: I bring a cup of water to a boil, add a generous amount of baking soda, stir it, pour it in, and close the drain for fifteen minutes.

I find I can no longer tolerate the fumes of most toilet bowl cleaners. I dip a cleaning rag in hot water, pour on some dry baking soda, and use that on the bowl itself. To clean inside the edges, I pour dry baking soda on a wet toilet brush and use that. It cleans fairly well, and deodorizes as well.

Before I conclude this chapter, I just want to caution you that if you do find an herbal remedy that works for you, it is not to be used forever, just as a medicine is not meant to be used forever. Use only when you have symptoms.

Also, if you are taking medicines, you should not take herbs. Herbs help the body by means of natural substances, whereas medicines and prescriptions are chemical, and the two don't mix.

That wraps up what I have to share with you regarding my experiences with home and herbal remedies.

CHAPTER XI

Stress Management and Time Management

Men and women today are subject to stress on all sides. It's dog eat dog out there in the working world. It's violence and disasters on the evening news. It's worry about children and drugs.

Families, once a center of stability and support, are instead yet another source of stress. The automobile gave us personal mobility, but it also provided the means for everyone to drive off in different directions, doing their own thing, subverting efforts to establish closeness within the family.

Today we have the nuclear family which many experts say imposes tremendous stress on its members. The parents are looked to for everything, instead of spreading the load among grandparents, aunts, uncles and cousins. The wife and mother, who once stayed home and baked the bread, must now go out and earn it, then come home and toast it.

A recent advertisement for a book on "wellness" began this way:

"Did you know that 75 per cent of all medical disorders are now believed to be related to stress?"

Yes, I know it now, and I can see how it led to my having cancer. The last five years that I worked were extremely stressful.

So, like many people do today, I went to several stress seminars. I was pleased to see many men in these classes. It was nice to know they had abandoned the strong, silent pose and were seeking help for their problems. I learned some good techniques, plus I developed some of my own as time went by. I will share them with you in the hope that you may find some of them helpful.

Bear in mind that stress seminars are all-day affairs, calling for intense personal involvement and are by no means easy. I learned that quite often it is a real struggle to give up fixed patterns of behavior. They may be self-defeating but they are all we know and in some peculiar way they have the comfort of being familiar.

We hesitate to stand up to a boss or a co-worker, for example. If we stand up to them, we are doing something different, which is unfamiliar and scary. And risky! We need to learn a very special kind of self-assertiveness for this sort of ticklish situation.

You may have to make drastic changes in your life. You may have to quit your job and find another. You may have to divorce your spouse. You may have to move away from difficult parents or relatives. It may take time to get up the courage to take such big steps, but if you must, you must.

If you are having teen-age family problems, here is an effective technique which I learned from a friend. I believe she said she learned it from Parent Effectiveness Training (PET).

Sit down with the kids (all of them, not just the troublemakers). Each person gets a piece of paper, including parents. Fold the paper in half, lengthwise. In the left-hand column, ask everyone to write down their rights. In the right-hand column, ask them to write down their responsibilities. Since THEY have thought them up, they are far more prone to live up to them.

Based on the above responsibilities, everyone writes up a

contract which they sign. Everyone (including parents) agrees to do certain things; if not, they face certain consequences, which are included in the contract.

IMPORTANT: They must be called CONSEQUENCES, not penalties or punishment.

Once again, since THEY have thought them up, they are far more prone to accept the consequences with good grace.

This is not an easy process. It may take several Saturday afternoons to work this out. There may be back-sliding. Renegotiation may often be necessary. But it can be very helpful. Just be sure to get the word PUNISHMENT out of your vocabulary when talking to your children. Replace it with CONSEQUENCES.

Assertiveness Training is also good. When I attended my first class, I was again pleased to see a fair number of men there. One thing leads to another and I found myself going to an Anger Seminar. This was very helpful also.

Many times I was angry about something but didn't even know it. For years I had the typical feminine habit of wanting to keep the peace, of wanting to make things pleasant for everybody.

I discovered I was afraid to express my anger for three basic reasons:

1) I was afraid it would draw anger in return

2) I was afraid I would expose myself and thus be vulnerable

3) I was angry with myself for failing in my duties

As for the first, when I finally gathered up my courage and expressed my anger, it did not always draw anger in return; often it drew surprise and an offer to change on the part of the other person.

It was a slow, difficult process, but I learned to express my anger to the person involved on the spot.

I learned to make "I" statements, such as:

I don't like it when you do (that). It makes me feel (whatever).

The first time I said it to anyone, I was quivering in my boots. The other person frowned, looked surprised, and said, Well, uh? Okay, I won't do it anymore. I was amazed.

I learned to come home from work, drop my purse on the table, put on walking shoes, and dash out the door for a vigorous walk.

I learned to go in the bedroom, shut the door, and punch the side of the mattress while cussing out the person or thing I was upset about.

This last always made me feel silly, but it did relieve my feelings.

Another thing I was doing, quite unconsciously, was putting myself down. I would say things like,

—Oh, I can't understand mutual funds

—Oh, I could never do that

—Oh, that book is too hard for me to read.

The teacher from the Anger Seminar gave us three helpful phrases to remember:

It is never too late (to change yourself, to correct a situation)

You did the best you could (when your kids go wild)

Forgive yourself for not doing a perfect job.

A middle-aged man in the Anger Seminar said he was secretly angry with his wife for always looking up to him and expecting him to make all the major decisions. Our teacher remarked, Yes, it is unfortunate that our society puts a man in the Top Dog position and expects him to function perfectly.

Another helpful thing our teacher told us was—KEEP YOUR FEELINGS CURRENT. When you hide your anger, your mind knows it is there and responds with emotional reactions like depression, anxiety, sexual impotence, frigidity. It also responds with physical symptoms like headaches, fatigue, ulcers, colitis.

A good technique for younger families is once a week or so, everyone gets together and is given three or five minutes each to air what is bothering them. They are not to attack others, they are to REPORT their feelings. Others listen but do not reply.

After this, it is time for appreciation. Everyone must say at least one thing they appreciate about someone else, or what the family is doing for them.

As for marital relationships, here are things I have discovered about managing men. I am sure they would work for women as well!

Give your spouse a sincere compliment every other day. It may have to do with something very tiny, but it must be sincere. Keep looking until you find something!

The days in between, give him or her an affectionate touch—outside the bedroom.

These two things combined do wonders for grouchy, stubborn spouses. When spouses are regularly told they are wonderful, after a while they become wonderful.

When serious differences arise, don't meet them head on. Slide into the topic side-wise. Try to get—and be satisfied with—a little bit of what you want. Don't be bull-headed. Don't expect to get your own way all the time. If you have a need to be right all the time, and win all the arguments, RUN, don't walk, to the nearest counselor. Marriage is a fifty-fifty proposition.

And here is a phrase from the Bible that is very helpful. Even the atheists among you will quickly see the usefulness of this advice:

LET ALL YOUR UTTERANCES BE GRACIOUS

If your spouse has a sore spot — a physical trait or a habit he or she is touchy about — stay off it. I repeat — stay off it.

If, on the other hand, your spouse gets on your sore spot and stays on it, say, "Yes, you're right, dear, I will try to correct it." This is a real defuser. Takes all the wind right out of their sails.

Then, privately, think about it. Maybe the other person is right. Who among us is perfect? Maybe you could improve on that point.

(The above advice does not necessarily apply if your spouse is addicted to alcohol or drugs. Alcoholic spouses in particular are past masters at blaming THEIR drinking on other people. The spouse of an alcoholic must avoid this trap.)

There is a power struggle that goes on in a great many marriages, with each spouse wanting his own way. This struggle must be settled if you are to have any peace.

The old days, when the woman ruled the house and the man earned the money and made the financial decisions, weren't all bad. Each knew his role and if both partners were mature and secure in themselves, things worked out just fine. Today, though, things are much more fluid.

In some marriages, it is helpful to have certain areas in which one spouse is boss, and certain areas for the other spouse to be boss. Tacit agreement is reached and harmony reigns.

In other marriages, as new issues come up, the power struggle surfaces and has to be decided every time. When both spouses have strong personalities, this occurs often. I understand that today in younger marriages the husbands are more agreeable to this constant renegotiation — largely because their young wives expect it. What works, works, and cannot be argued with.

For both spouses, it is very helpful to have support systems. This means friends or relatives you can TALK to freely.

Keeping feelings inside you is more stressful than unloading them. If you have no friends, sign up for an Assertiveness Training course or Stress Seminar. As you become more relaxed and sure of yourself, you will attract friends in whom you can confide.

Develop your sense of humor. Get funny books from the library. If you can't change things, make jokes about them. It may be black humor, but you must get your laughs however you can.

Humor helps with children, too. When my boys were teen-agers and their rooms got messy, I'd say, It looks like fifteen pink elephants have been rampaging in here. They'd laugh but it made them realize their rooms were messy and they'd pick up.

Another thing that can be very helpful in relieving stress is Yoga. I began practicing Yoga as a lark in the late 1960's and enjoyed the increased circulation and loosening up of joints. After doing it for a year, I realized that gradually many of my hostilities and irritabilities had vanished and I had a much more relaxed attitude toward life in general. If I had to wait in line, for instance, it didn't bother me.

The sad thing about Yoga in this country is that relatively few men practice it. I think it's because it so happens that most books written about Yoga feature mainly photos of women performing the postures, and men who see these books automatically think Yoga is for women.

Also, classes are usually offered during the day and men can't attend because they are at work. Last year I attended a Yoga Day which took place on Saturday and there were ten men in attendance out of a total of about eighty students. I noticed the men all had very nice builds, regardless of their age. That is to say, no bellies hanging over their belts.

What is commonly practiced in America is Hatha Yoga and it does not involve any mysticism or religious elements. It involves exercising the body. But I must immediately correct that and be more specific.

Yoga involves POSTURES, not mere exercise. It is not doing twenty jumping jacks and twenty push-ups and then being exhausted and stiff as a board the next day. You do warm-ups, then you slowly stretch your body into a posture, hold it, and come out of it slowly and with control. If you do the exercises properly, you will NEVER be stiff the next day.

Yoga postures emphasize the breath. Usually you inhale as you go up and exhale as you go down. Yoga postures stretch and flex the spine, muscles, nerves AND massage the internal organs, thus promoting proper elimination, blood circulation, and gland function. It is highly recommended for people with arthritis of the spine because the slow, gentle movements enable the person to keep moving.

Yoga classes are not expensive and do not require elaborate equipment. They are available in most communities.

TIME MANAGEMENT

This is a serious problem for everyone these days. We all have plenty of chores and errands to do, plus there are so many activities and forms of entertainment to entice us and take up our time. There are dozens of periodicals we would like to read, either for entertainment or for information. Many interesting new books are being published. All this on top of our jobs and our basic daily routines.

As a working mother I felt the time crunch very severely. I had to go to work, come home and get the meals, and take care of my children and house as well. I also was trying to squeeze out some time for my writing.

In the years immediately after the onset of my cancer, after I quit work and stayed home, my raw vegetable diet led to continuing "healing crises" which reduced my store of energy to zero. I couldn't do anything about my time problem for a long period until my health improved, but I utilized those years by clipping cancer and general medical articles and saving them.

Here are my suggestions on time management, gleaned from many sources and passed through the crucible of my personal experience. It was a question of trial and error. Some things didn't work because they didn't apply to my situation. Some didn't work because they didn't suit my personality. It will be trial and error for you, too, but I hope my suggestions will be of some help to you.

If you are a person who doesn't like to write things down, you can probably do just as well by thinking about them carefully, although if you could manage to scribble down a few words it would be helpful.

Develop time awareness:
   What do you want time for?
   What wastes your time?
   What are you forced to spend time on?
After you've thought about these things for a week or so, here is the next step.
Develop awareness of what you really want time for:
   Do you want more schooling so you can get a better job?
   Do you want to see Paris?
   Do you want to compete in a marathon running race?
   Do you want _____?

Try to be specific in your answers. Don't say I want to be happy. Rather, say I want to earn more money by learning more. Or, I want less friction around the house.

Now let's talk about how much time there is. There are 168 hours in the week. Deduct 56 hours for seven nights' sleep. This leaves 112 hours for your job, commuting to it, eating your meals, and other essentials. I have gone through this with many friends, and it usually comes out to 29 hours a week left for all other things such as . . .

Taking out the garbage, clearing snow, playing with your children, getting gas, mowing the lawn, doing the laundry, purchasing groceries, watching television, reading magazines . . . and I haven't even mentioned cleaning house.

So it is easy to see why everyone suffers a time crunch.
One of the techniques I rely heavily on is the making of lists. I make a weekly list, divided into days, anticipating appointments and errands. I do this whenever the need strikes. I usually make a list for each day, sometimes in the morning. Though sometimes at night, if I can't sleep because there are too many activities looming ahead, I get up and make a list for the next day.

I also keep a perennial shopping list in my purse, for clothing, cosmetics or other items. I include sizes and other details. Then if I am doing errands and find myself near a shopping mall I can easily look at the list and see what I need. I don't have to rack my brain wondering what I might need.

Above all, I try to be flexible about making lists. I don't do them at specified times, just when the need strikes. If I don't get it all done, I don't bemoan the fact. I just say, next time will be fine.

For the housewife, may I remind her of the old saying, "Many hands make light work." Get your family to help with household chores. Start while the children are young and be relentless about making them follow through.

If they are teen-agers and lazy and/or rebellious, work chores into the contracts you make with them, as outlined earlier. No chores, no allowance. Or, no chores, no privileges. Important Point: be sure to pick a privilege that means a lot to them.

Keeping things picked up as you go along is very helpful. Wife off fingerprints before they set in. Vacuum up spills before they are ground in. Make your bed when you get out of it. Wash dishes right after eating. Hang up your clothes when you take them off.

Organize your chores and get on top of them. Do the ones that show the most. Clean out the cabinets only when they scream to be cleaned, and get someone else to help. Plan a nice treat for you both when the beastly job is done.

Schedule some "down time" for yourself.

Many husbands and wives are frantically busy on weekends catching up on errands and chores. If you get to feeling too pressured, just flop down on a comfortable chair, or on the floor. Close your eyes, mentally put your worries in a box behind you, and for five minutes imagine that you are sunning yourself on a tropical beach. Concentrate on your breathing, and bring it into unison with the waves, which are lapping gently on the beach.

Here are a few hints on household management that I have found helpful. They might also come under the heading of saving steps.

Keep duplicate scissors, rolls of cellophane tape, boxes of facial tissue, pens and paper, in places where they are urgently needed. The idea here is to keep things at the POINT OF USE.

Keep a small mending kit near the washer for last minute repairs.

Keep several threaded needles ready in the pin cushion in your bedroom; white thread for last-minute lingerie rescues, beige for stockings, and no-color for everything else.

Keep duplicate cleaning supplies in both bathroom and kitchen. When cleaning house, put one set in a garden caddy and carry it around with you.

Think about litter and how to avoid it. Litter means things left out after use. It means things sitting on top of dressers and tables that should be put away. One of the biggest time consumers in cleaning house is picking up litter and putting it away. In fact, when you clean a room, buzz around picking up all the litter first, then the cleaning itself will go faster.

If you have a small house with little storage space, you have a serious problem. What you can do is (1) throw things out as often as possible and (2) organize your closets. Nowadays there are closet clutter shops that sell useful bins and racks to make storage more efficient.

In general, out of sight, out of mind. Try to have a place to keep all the daily newspapers out of sight. Clear off the tops of furniture and a neat look will be achieved instantly.

I used to make a big mistake by resenting the time I spent planning. Finally I realized that time spent planning is time well spent. It helps you gain control and feel competent and efficient. Many women tend to feel helpless and one way this manifests itself is acting as if they are not strong enough to take control of their household routine.

I know a young woman whose mother refuses to visit her anymore because her house is dirty and sloppy. When they argue about it, the young woman says, You know I don't like housework. My answer to that is: WHO DOES? No one likes housework, but most women do it because it has to be done, and because it is far more pleasant to live in a clean, neat house where you can find things when you need them.

If you are disorganized, first, decide to change, and second, use behavior modification to change yourself. Choose a reward that is meaningful to you and reward yourself.

Behavior modification began years ago with experiments with retarded children, as attempts were made to help them learn some basic self-care. Every action was broken down into little parts. Every time the child did one little part correctly, he was given one piece of candy. It was a very small button-shaped chocolate candy with a hard coating.

You might try popping one of these candies in your mouth occasionally as you improve. Then later on when your house is ship-shape and your life is organized, your feeling of being competent and in control will be reward enough. You may not need the candy.

FOOTNOTE TO YOUNG MOTHERS: If you are a mother with a new baby, here are a few general tips.

Feed the baby first, so he doesn't cry. Demand feeding is all right, but I think it's better to get him on a schedule as quickly as possible. If you know you will be feeding him every three hours, or whatever, it makes it easier on you.

Breast feed as long as possible for his future health. PLEASE don't feed him commercial baby foods, they are full of artificial ingredients which set the baby up for a lifetime of being hooked on junk foods. To prepare pureed foods for your infant, simply take a little of your own food and whiz briefly in blender. If you don't have a blender, overcook his portion slightly until food is mushy and rub through a coarse sieve.

After feeding the baby, the next thing is the family's meals. Do the dishes right away.

Next comes a little time for your own personal grooming. Try to slick yourself up early in the day, you'll feel better.

Next comes laundry of baby clothes and diapers. Don't rely too heavily on disposable diapers; many bad cases of diaper rash result from their use. Save them for trips and other outings. Arrange for diaper service for the first six months, if possible.

Next comes time with your husband.

After that comes housecleaning. If you keep things picked up as you go along, and if you keep the living room slicked up and baby things elsewhere, the house will be a welcoming sight to your husband when he comes home in the evening.

Pay a little attention to your own nutritional needs. Eat fresh fruits, especially those which are in season; eat a lot of dark green lettuce in your salads. You probably need iron. There is a line of vitamins which offers "Organic Iron" derived from "elemental iron from Ferrous Fumarate" which is not constipating. Avoid junk foods, fast foods, and additives. If you are really hooked on them, try to cut back.

If your baby is a screamer, don't blame it on yourself. Some are just born that way. Remain calm yourself and he will respond favorably. You have produced a miracle, take pride in the dear little being.

CHAPTER XII

Is Cancer Big Business?

President Richard M. Nixon declared "war" on cancer during his term of office in the early 1970's.

As I write this, the improvement in the survival rate has been very small. Some experts says it is only 1 per cent.

I have heard people say, brutally, that cancer will never be cured because there is too much money in the business of treating it.

At the end of the book I have included photocopies of information from the American Cancer Society itself, from its official update of February, 1984.

Page three, Column 1, says: "870,000 people will be diagnosed as having cancer this year."

At a modest guess of $1,000 in medical costs for one year, 870,000 multiplied by $1,000 equals $870,000,000.

Page three, Column 2, says: "This year about 450,000 will die of the disease."

Figuring an average of $30,000 per person to die of cancer, this amounts to $13.5 billion.

Who gets this money?
Doctors. Drug companies. Hospitals.

The copy of an article which I've included from the Detroit News begins, "Harper Hospital will spend **$8.5 million** to buy and install a cyclotron designed to treat an assortment of normally fatal cancers with powerfully built neutron radiation."

I leave it up to you to decide whether cancer is big business.

* * * *

What did it cost me to conquer cancer?

To repeat what I said in Chapter Five—in the beginning it cost me $140 for a juicer and $80 for a blender. Since then it has cost me $20 a week for vegetables.

(I have saved thousands on meat over the past ten years.)

CANCER FACTS & FIGURES

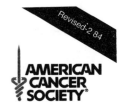
Revised-2 84

AMERICAN CANCER SOCIETY®

1984

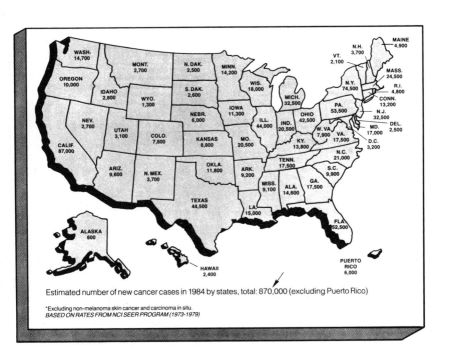

WASH. 14,700	MAINE 4,900
MONT. 2,700	N.H. 3,700
N. DAK. 2,500	VT. 2,100
MINN. 14,200	MASS. 24,500
OREGON 10,000	N.Y. 74,500
IDAHO 2,800	R.I. 4,800
S. DAK. 2,600	CONN. 13,200
WYO. 1,300	MICH. 32,500
WIS. 18,000	PA. 53,500
NEBR. 6,000	N.J. 32,500
IOWA 11,300	OHIO 42,500
NEV. 2,700	DEL. 2,500
ILL. 44,000	IND. 20,500
UTAH 3,100	W. VA 7,900
COLO. 7,800	VA. 17,500
MD. 17,000	D.C. 3,200
CALIF. 87,000	KANSAS 8,800
MO. 20,500	KY. 13,800
N.C. 21,000	ARIZ. 9,600
N. MEX. 3,700	OKLA. 11,800
TENN. 17,500	S.C. 9,900
ARK. 9,200	GA. 17,500
MISS. 9,100	ALA. 14,600
TEXAS 44,500	LA. 15,000
FLA. 52,500	ALASKA 600
HAWAII 2,400	PUERTO RICO 6,000

Estimated number of new cancer cases in 1984 by states, total: 870,000 (excluding Puerto Rico)

*Excluding non-melanoma skin cancer and carcinoma in situ.
BASED ON RATES FROM NCI SEER PROGRAM (1973-1979)

the cyclotron: how it attacks cancer

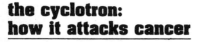

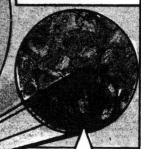

Advantage of neutron therapy over X-rays is that neutron therapy causes *less damage* to healthy cells.

1. Atomic nuclei between magnetic poles are set into motion by electrical jolts. Magnetic fields of poles act like banked ends on a race track, forcing particles into a circular pattern. (At full power, poles pull against each other with a force of about 150 tons.)

Cylindrical electromagnetic poles 26 inches in diameter and separated by one inch.

2. Particle speed increases (up to 42,000 miles per second) and orbit widens until particles hit "target" of beryllium or substance maximizing neutron production.

3. The particles' collisions with the target "smashes" the atoms. The neutrons are released and directed toward the cells to be treated.

Source: Cyclotron Laboratory, Michigan State University

Free Press Graphic by MARTHA THIERRY

Harper Hospital to get cancer-fighting cyclotron

By JOHN FLYNN
Free Press Staff Writer

Harper Hospital will spend $8.5 million to buy and install a cyclotron designed to treat an assortment of normally fatal cancers with powerfully beamed neutron radiation.

Hospital officials suggest that the 23-ton machine, to be designed and constructed by Michigan State University in partnership with Harper and two private firms, will propel the hospital into a national leadership role in cancer treatment.

Plans to buy the cyclotron, which should be in operation by late 1986, were announced Wednesday by Harper officials.

The $1.5 million radiation unit will be the first of its kind, though heavier and more expensive modern neutron units are in use in Seattle and Houston.

See **CYCLOTRON**, Page 17A

CHAPTER XIII

Be Your Own Best Expert

As I look over my files as I near completion of this book, I am amazed at the wealth of information I have collected. I have a stack of clippings about four inches high, divided into six folders.

As I look at the list of books I have read — many of them at one time far beyond my comprehension — I am amazed at how much I have learned. My mind has stretched more than I ever thought it would.

I am convinced the average cancer patient needs to become his own expert on health.

For example, if I had listened to the surgeon who wanted to operate, at this moment I would be missing a breast. I might even be dead. Of ten people I know who had cancer, who chose conventional treatment, seven are dead.

But I said "No," to that surgeon and searched out an alternative method.

Not only the average cancer patient needs to become his own expert, the average person needs to do the same thing.

As good as your doctor may be, he will never KNOW your body, its feelings, its reactions to drugs, the way you do.

There is no "mystique" about one's body. If a doctor can learn, limb by limb and gland by gland, with lots of review and repetition, so can we. All we have to do is make up our mind to do it.

I think it is happening. Everywhere in the United States today people are taking more responsibility for their health. They are getting into fitness and more and more into "health foods."

On the radio recently I heard an announcement that a survey found that more than half the people felt a correct diet can prevent illness, INCLUDING cancer.

It is only a step to the belief that correct diet can CURE illness, including cancer.

In fact, more and more medical doctors are publishing books that are not entirely in line with the "drug them and cut them" ideas of the American Medical Association. Some of these are, Dr. Cooper, Dr. MacDougall, Dr. Sattilaro, and Dr. Atkins.

I urge you to become your own best expert. You can do it! When something puzzles you, study it. Begin your studies in the Children's Section of your local public library.

There are some remarkably well-written informative books in that section. Books for children must be very honest because children won't put up with anything else.

Books for children must measure up to the standards not only of the writer and his editor, but also of the librarian and the teacher. Once a book as passed all these hurdles, it is truly a good book, with accurate information. It also has the benefit of being clear and easy to read. I'm thinking chiefly of books for age 10 and up. Biology, anatomy, and physiology are made simple and easy to understand. The encyclopedias for juniors are also helpful, and are the best place to start.

Let us talk now about articles in newspapers and magazines. As you read these, you must be aware of WHO the writer is. What is his slant? Where is he or she coming from? I regret to say that some big-name health writers in this country are virtually in the pay of the American Medical Association (AMA).

The AMA offers a big cash prize and a trip to Florida

every year to the writer who does the "best science writing." Meaning, of course, writing that is totally in line with the ideas of the AMA, which I think you will agree boil down to "drug them and cut them." Writers will not be rewarded for telling you about alternatives.

Also, be aware of WHERE the article appears. The top women's magazines are firmly wedded to the idea that the men in white are HEROES who labor ceaselessly to come up with new methods to SAVE us. The new methods always involve tests and drugs that line the pockets of drug companies or equipment manufacturers.

If the magazine carries advertisements for over-the-counter medicines, you can be sure the mind-set of the writers will see nothing wrong in subtly or actively urging you to pop those pills.

If it is a health magazine with advertisements for vitamin supplements, you may be sure vitamin tablets rather than raw foods will be recommended.

With regard to the daily paper, be aware that newspaper reporters work in a severe time crunch with deadlines looming over their heads. They don't always have the time to think things through fully and you may get only part of the story.

Be aware that sometimes, even if the article is written correctly, paragraphs may be cut out at random. Why? To make room for advertisements! This explains why some newspaper articles don't really make sense—something important has been cut out.

As you read, be skeptical. Be informed. Be your own best expert.

You CAN do it!

As Dr. Goldstein says in his wonderful book, "The mind is like a parachute—it only functions when open."

Open up your mind, and fly!

Postscript 1

It is now ten years later, and you may ask me, "Do you still maintain the diet?"

Yes, I do. The few times that I added too many impure foods, I'd have a relapse, so I follow it very closely. I eat about 50 per cent raw food. In the form of vegetable juice, it is readily assimilated by the intestines and goes right to work cleansing and nourishing.

You may ask me, "Do you think you are recovered?"

Yes, I do. I do all my own housework. I work at my writing four days a week. I have a rose garden and a vegetable garden and except for the heavy work in spring, do most of the work myself. I go on lengthy trips with my husband. My sons are good citizens, hard working and ambitious. Most of the time I feel cheerful and energetic.

Could I ask for anything more? Yes, two breasts — and that is what I have — because I drastically changed my eating habits. It was a miracle, a miracle of my own body, accomplished by my immune system.

Postscript 2

I want to share with you another success story attributable to raw vegetable diet.

In July of 1984, my mother-in-law, Vera, had been living with us about six years. She had reached the age of 86 and was becoming increasingly infirm, and her care was getting to be too much for us. Dave decided that she should move to a nursing home, and a family discussion was held. At first she refused to leave and made a terrible scene. Dave kept explaining things to her and she finally agreed.

On the day she actually left, she changed her mind and created another terrible scene over breakfast. Dave felt awful. He loved her dearly and was very devoted to her. He hated to have her leave, but she was falling down a great deal and the worry was too much. He prevailed, telling her it would be like a hotel with room service. The home provided especially large bathrooms with wide doors. She could get through the doors easily with her walker, and there would be a toilet with big handles on the side so she could maneuver more easily. In the end, lady that she is, she left graciously.

Soon afterward Dave went into a tailspin. He began suffering severe spells of dizziness and didn't dare drive a car. A few months earlier he had been having pains in the back, as if from gall bladder, and they intensified. The previous April he had begun having prostate trouble; an enlargement had been found and an operation had been recommended. He had been putting off this decision.

Now, however, his dizzy spells were the big worry. He was

sent for a glucose tolerance test, which yielded the fact that he was borderline diabetic. He went for a battery of neurological tests which, fortunately, came out negative.

With regard to the gall bladder, he underwent ultra sound tests which discovered small multiple stones.

It is my personal opinion that Dave's grief and guilt over having his mother leave us worsened the symptoms he had and led to the dizziness. Dave brushes this aside and says it all just happened coincidentally.

Be that as it may, two operations were recommended — one for the prostate enlargement, and one for the gallstones.

Dave thought about it, then said, "If my wife can lick cancer with a change in diet, maybe I can avoid these operations the same way."

So, on August 29th, 1984, Dave began a raw juice diet. He consulted Dr. Walker's book RAW VEGETABLE JUICES, and decided on a regimen. Before breakfast he drank the juice of half a lemon with enough hot water added to yield a cupful. After a while, he increased this to the juice of a whole lemon. Three times a day he drank a mixture of raw carrot juice, beet juice, and cucumber juice. He also eliminated carbohydrates from his diet.

This last was difficult for him, since he had the habit of snacking on cookies and ice cream during the evening. But motivated as he was by the desire to avoid two operations, he managed to give up his evening treats.

Six weeks after changing his diet he noticed an improvement in his condition. As time went by his health continued to improve, and at this writing, he has no symptoms and has not needed the operations. So, you see, another victory for raw vegetable diet.

Questions I am Often Asked

Why does a person get cancer?

Dr. Harold Manner, head of Biology Dept. at Loyola University (now retired) says everyone gets cancer about once a week because our food is so adulterated and our environment so polluted, but one's immune system routinely vanquishes it.

However, when the immune system is low, which can occur for a variety of reasons, it cannot vanquish cancer (or other diseases which are lying in wait).

How and why does raw diet work?

It restores the correct metabolic balance within the body, allowing the immune system to kick in and attack the cancer cells.

Has this diet helped people with other ailments?

Margie Garrison was cured of a severe case of arthritis. She wrote a book about her experience (see Reading List.) Margie has graciously served as my mentor while I wrote this book.

Ed Wolfrum, whose kidneys were in such bad shape that Mayo Clinic refused to take him, was helped to the point where he was able to fly off to Japan on a business trip.

(Mayo Clinic is a complex of buildings containing many specialists who are very up-to-date. They ask for your complete medical records. If they don't think they can help you, they will not accept you. A refusal from them sometimes amounts to a death sentence.)

What about Laetrile?

The AMA is determined that Laetrile be labelled as being worthless. Laetrile, also called amygdalin, is B-17, which is a vitamin, which is a food stuff, which is NOT PATENT-ABLE. Therefore, there is no fortune in it for doctors, pharmacists, or drug companies.

Has Laetrile been successful?

Yes. Dr. Richardson, Dr. Contreras and others have had success with it. Dr. Richardson of California, who used it on terminally ill cases and saved them, was brutally hounded out of the state by the California AMA.

How is Laetrile given when used properly?

Dr. Manner's lab experiments have shown that when used alone, Laetrile is useless. When used with other things, it is useless unless administered at the proper time.

When a tumor gets started, after a short time it throws up a shield to protect itself from the immune system, which, recognizing it as a foreign body, will dissolve it. When this shield (fibrin) is established it must be dissolved by (1) enzymes (2) colonics (3) natural diet and THEN when the doctor determines it has been dissolved, Laetrile is given and will vanquish the cancer cells. The foregoing is the method devised by Dr. Manner. It must be done in a clinic away from home (so that you are away from the stresses of your life) and is very expensive. Some insurance companies cover it. Among others, it saved a man whose prostrate cancer was so bad he couldn't climb steps.

Why is the conventional medical approach wrong?

It fights cancer as if it is caused by something OUTSIDE the body, WHEREAS CANCER IS CAUSED by something going wrong INSIDE the body.

Chemotherapy and radiation kill many normal cells along with cancer cells. Medical doctors know this, but their hope is that the body is strong enough to withstand this onslaught.

Is there any money in curing cancer the conventional way?

I have in hand a bulletin from the American Cancer Society itself, giving figures for 1984. This OFFICIAL update, page three, column 2, says, "This year about 450,000 will die of the disease."

Figuring an average of $30,000 per person to die of cancer, this amounts to $13.5 billion. Who gets this money?

DOCTORS. DRUG COMPANIES. HOSPITALS.

What did it cost Louise Greenfield to overcome her cancer?

It cost her $120 for a juicer, $80 for a heavy duty blender, and $20 a week for vegetables. She saved thousands of dollars on meat.

Are there occasions when surgery might be recommended?

Yes, when the cancerous growth is blocking a vital passageway.

What is the Natural Hygiene Society about?

It is a non-profit organization dedicated to educating the public about correct eating. They are against meat, milk and too much cooked food. They stress fresh fruits and vegetables, food combining, (eating foods in certain combinations which permit more efficient digestion in the intestines) and trying to achieve "emotional poise." They believe a person should strive for a lifestyle stressing natural diet, fresh air, pure water, proper rest, exercise, and essential calmness towards life's troubles.

Why is Louise Greenfield writing a book about her experience?

As Mrs. Jack Goldstein has said, there have been too many books written which make heroes out of women who go the conventional route, meekly allowing themselves to be mutilated, NOT EVEN KNOWING there is any alternative.

What is beneficial about Yoga?

It reduces irritabilities and hostilities. It calms the body and the mind. It improves concentration. Yoga involves breath control and slow, graceful postures. It considers the health of the spine essential. Yoga postures stretch and flex the spine, and at the same time, they tone up muscles, nerves, and massage the internal organs, thus promoting proper elimination, blood circulation, and gland function. It takes the "racing thoughts" out of your mind and allows you to concentrate on your body.

ANOTHER BONUS: YOGA SLOWS DOWN THE PROCESS OF AGING.

Since stress is one of the basic factors causing disease, Yoga, by calming both body and mind, is an important aid in conquering illness and/or keeping it away.

Is there a connection between Yoga and Chiropractic care?

Yes, they both emphasize the health and flexibility of the spine. All body activities are regulated by the nervous system which consists of the brain, the spinal cord and a farflung network of nerves. The spine is a vertical pathway for all the nerves which in turn give energy to all organs and parts of the body. Distortions of the spine lead to many problems. Cancer is an uncontrollable action of body cells. If the body is kept in optimum condition, cancer cells can't get started.

While I don't say keeping your spine healthy will vanquish cancer, I do know a healthy spine keeps you moving gracefully and youthfully. I personally have been greatly helped by regular chiropractic care. At one time I couldn't bend over to weed my garden; now I can work hours at a time. I have also witnessed the manner in which chiropractic extended my mother-in-law's life. I feel almost everyone could benefit from regular chiropractic adjustments, because the health of the spine is so crucial.

How does stress cause disease?

Stress causes the adrenal gland to over-function, and it sends extra hormone into the body; when this becomes excessive, the chemical balance of the body is thrown off, the immune system gets low, and it cannot do its job of attacking and getting rid of foreign bodies.

Why not simply eat the raw vegetables by themselves, saving the work of juicing and blending them?

There are three reasons why not. First, such an enormous quantity is required that it would be impossible to sit down long enough to eat them. Second, there would be gas, discomfort, and too much work for the digestive system. Third, when converted into raw juice, they go almost directly to the intestines and provide instant nourishment and elimination of toxins.

Have you been back to the doctor to make sure you don't have cancer?

No, I have no intentions of doing that because the tests he'd want to do would put poison into my system. One of the main things I want to do is keep chemicals out of my body. As long as I don't have any lumps or other signs of cancer and can live a normal life, then I consider myself healthy and there is no need to go to a doctor and have him tell me what I already know.

What do you recommend as the most important things in keeping cancer away?

The first and most important thing is keeping chemicals out of your body. That means eating pure food and avoiding drugs. Second, learn to handle the stress in your life constructively, on a daily basis. Strive for "emotional poise". Don't let bad feelings pile up. Have a quiet time every day.

None of the above is easy. Health is an on-going, do-it-yourself process. YOU must work at it, and YOU will reap the rewards.

This book is the story of my personal struggle with cancer and the unique method I chose to overcome it. My book is not intended to replace the advice of your doctor.

Publisher's Note: *Photograph on back cover was taken in November, 1985.*

Comments From a Critic
Within the Medical Profession

In some medical circles the New England Journal of Medicine is considered to be more prestigious and more scholarly than the Journal of the American Medical Association. In the May 8, 1986 issue of the NEJM there appeared an article by Dr. John C. Bailor and Elaine M. Smith. Dr. Bailor entered the field of cancer research 25 years ago, as an enthusiastic young researcher, at a time when they were saying the cure to cancer was "just around the corner." When his article was published he was invited to appear on national television. He said frankly that he was disillusioned because the cure is still "just around the corner." He declared there must be a switch to prevention in research efforts and that the National Cancer Institute owes the American public an apology.

His article tells how mortality rates are based on figures drawn from death certificates, which figures have been adjusted carefully for shifts, changes and growth in population. It contains charts and tables which show that for some cancers there has been only a 1 per cent or 2 per cent improvement, whereas for other cancers the cure rate has decreased.

The title of Dr. Bailor's and Ms. Smith's article is very revealing: Progress against Cancer?

Later in the body of the article, on page 1228, the following paragraph appears:

"These data, taken alone, provide no evidence that some 35 years of intense and growing efforts to improve the treatment of cancer have had much overall effect on the most fundamental measure of clinical outcome — death. Indeed, with respect to cancer as a whole we have slowly lost ground, as shown by the rise in age-adjusted mortality rates in the entire population. This is not to say that without these efforts at treatment the trends would have been the same, but overall, the effort to control cancer has failed — so far — to attain its objectives."

In other words, the medical establishment's fight against cancer has been a losing battle.

Additional copies of this book may be obtained by sending $9.95 plus $1.00 (postage and handling) to Midwest Publishing Company, 19970 Lathers Avenue, Livonia, MI 48152.

SUGGESTED READING

Anatomy of an Illness, As Perceived by the Patient, Norman Cousins, 1979 W. W. Norton & Co., New York. Stricken by a mysterious illness and given little hope, Mr. Cousins studied the factors that lead to self-healing, devised his own regimen and saved his own life.

Born to Win: Transactional Analysis with Gestalt Experiments, by Muriel James and Dorothy Jongeward, Addison-Wesley Publishing Co., Reading, MA, 1971. A landmark book. Don't let the sub-title scare you off. It's thoroughly readable and very helpful to the average person in learning to understand and modify behavior.

A Consumer's Dictionary of Food Additives by Ruth Winter, Crown Publishers, New York, 1984. Paperback. Very detailed. Its introduction must be read carefully to get full value from the book. Describes additives, gives uses and whether toxic or not. Based on rulings of the FDA.

Fit for Life, by Harvey and Marilyn Diamond, Warner Books, 1985. Big best seller of 1985 and 1986 for 66 weeks. Lively and well-written, it gives a program for weight loss and fitness based on the principles of the Natural Hygiene Society, the same as those used by Dr. Goldstein for my diet.

I Cured my Arthritis, You Can Too, by Margie Garrison, Uptown Publishers, Wyandotte, MI, 1980. Chatty account of author's brush with osteoarthritis and how years of conventional treatment led only to huge doses of painkillers. Margie sought nutritional counseling from Dr. Goldstein and cured herself. Menus, recipes, exercises.

Natural Hygiene Society, 12816 Racetrack Road, Tampa, FL 33625. Write for list of current publications.

The Politics of Cancer, by Samuel S. Epstein, M.D., Sierra Club Books, 1978. A big book, rather technical, written by a professor of occupational and environmental medicine with many years' experience in toxicology and ecology. Explains how many scientific decisions are influenced by economics, and concludes that the public faces a real threat from the medical-industrial complex.

Raw, Vegetable Juices, by Dr. N. W. Walker, Norwalk Press, Phoenix, AZ, 1936 and many further editions. Paperback. Discusses enzymes as vital nutrients and why raw vegetable juices are superior in providing them. Lists juice formulas for many ailments. Can be found in health food stores.

The Stress of Life by Dr. Hans Selye, McGraw-Hill, New York, 1956. Trail-blazing work by the grandfather of stress, whose experiments isolated it, defined it, and named it.

Triumph Over Disease by Fasting and Natural Diet, Dr. Jack Goldstein, Arco Publishing, New York, 1977. Dr. Goldstein's account of how he cured himself of a devastating case of ulcerative colitis reads like an adventure story. He includes case histories, takes pokes at the medical profession, tells why fad diets are useless, and explains natural living.

You Are What You Want to To Be, by Dr. L. N. Yuille, 1986, Metro Holistic Health Center, P.O. Box 866, Southfield, MI 48037. A family practitioner, Dr. Yuille came to see that stress is a primary cause of disease and switched to psychological counseling. Though having relatively little text, it is delightfully poetic and makes you see that you are where you are because you've made many choices along the way. The insight comes that, if you want to, you can make new choices and be somewhere better. Not available in bookstores. Send money order for $5.95 plus $1.00 for postage and handling to the publisher.

Index